Health-related behaviour and attitudes of older people:

a secondary analysis of national datasets

Health-related behaviour and attitudes of older people:

a secondary analysis of national datasets

Helen Cooper, Jay Ginn and Sara Arber
Institute of Social Research, Department of Sociology, University of Surrey

Acknowledgements

The Health Education Authority would like to thank the authors, Helen Cooper, Jay Ginn and Sara Arber, from the Department of Sociology, University of Surrey, for having carried out this project. Thanks are also due to Christine Callum, the Data Archive and Manchester Computing Services, for access to the datasets used in this report.

Authors of this report

Helen Cooper, *Research Fellow, University of Surrey*
Jay Ginn, *Research Fellow, University of Surrey*
Sara Arber, *Professor of Sociology, University of Surrey*

HEA Research Project Team

Seta Waller, *Research Manager*
Dominic McVey, *Head of Research*
Adam Crosier, *Senior Researcher*

ISBN 0 7521 1449 2

First published 1999

Health Education Authority
Trevelyan House
30 Great Peter Street
London SW1P 2HW

Text composition Ken Brooks
Printed in Great Britain

Contents

Foreword

The health of older people has sometimes been treated as less important than that of younger people, either because older people are considered less productive or because ill health is deemed an inevitable consequence of later life. Furthermore, older people are often regarded as a homogeneous group, which in turn conceals inequalities in this population. With these issues in mind the HEA commissioned a number of research projects to highlight the diversity of older people's health needs and the health promotion issues relevant to later life. The first of these studies published by the HEA was a review entitled *Researching older people's health needs and health promotion issues*, and it examined the influence of the physical and social environment on older people's health and highlighted gaps in the current research literature. The third project was a qualitative study entitled *Assessing older people's health and social needs*, which looked in detail at the social factors influencing health beliefs and health promoting behaviour. The results of the second project *Health-related behaviour and attitudes of older people – a secondary analysis of national datasets* are presented in this report. This work goes beyond the basic descriptive analysis provided by many large-scale government surveys to look deeper into the data and examine the diversity within older populations. Four British datasets have been subjected to multivariate analysis looking at a range of issues including diet, smoking, alcohol consumption and physical activity to identify the characteristics shared by those most likely to engage in health damaging behaviour.

All those concerned with the health and well being of older people will find in this report fresh and valuable insights into this diverse, under-researched and increasingly important population.

Dominic McVey
Head of Research
Health Education Authority

Executive summary

1. There has previously been a lack of research on older people's health-related behaviour. This report analyses four types of health-related behaviour, namely smoking, drinking, diet and physical activity among older people aged 55 and over, using three national surveys: the Health Survey for England (1993 and 1994), the General Household Survey (1992–4) and the Health Education and Monitoring Survey (1995 and 1996).
2. With increasing age, older men and women are less likely to eat a healthy diet and be physically active, and are more likely to be fatalistic about health. However, levels of smoking and drinking decrease with advancing age, with presumed health benefits.
3. Older women are less likely to smoke and drink than older men, and are more likely to have a healthy diet, but levels of physical activity are much lower for women than men in all older age groups.
4. Contrary to previous research, there is no strong evidence that increasingly fatalistic attitudes about health in later life can be attributed to the greater prevalence of chronic illness.
5. Poor health status is a major constraint on the physical activity of older men and women. There is a need for health promotion strategies which advocate increased physical activity while taking into account the differing levels of health, mobility and financial resources of older people.
6. Older men who are widowed or divorced are particularly likely to engage in health-damaging behaviour compared with married men. They are more likely to smoke, have a poor diet and report excessive levels of drinking. This group should be targeted in health promotion campaigns.
7. There is less difference between the health-related behaviour of older women according to their marital status, but single older women seem to exhibit the best health behaviour. Older married women have a higher alcohol intake, and widowed and divorced older women have higher levels of smoking.
8. Material circumstances have a crucial impact on health-related behaviour in later life. The major factors associated with older people smoking, having a poor diet and taking little physical activity are the class of their last occupation, living on a low income and living in more materially deprived circumstances. Health promotion strategies should address the ways in which social disadvantage handicaps older people in adopting a more healthy lifestyle.
9. Drinking amongst older people is associated with both material advantage and disadvantage. However, the highest levels of

excessive drinking are found among the most deprived and socially isolated men.

10. Social support is only associated in a minor way with health-related behaviour (smoking and diet) in comparison with the major effect of structural factors.
11. Older people with higher levels of educational qualification have less fatalistic attitudes about health, which suggests that later cohorts are likely to have attitudes which are more conducive to adopting health-promoting behaviours.

1 Introduction

Although chronological age is associated with increased risk of mortality, ill-health or functional disability (Martin, Meltzer and Elliot, 1988), this association with age can blind us to the diversity in health experience within particular age groups. Older people's health and involvement in health-promoting behaviour is influenced by their life course, in terms of their gender, occupation and employment history, housing and marital history. Differences within age groups may be more important than differences between age groups. The relative influence on health of structural variables and of individual behaviour has been the subject of extensive debate (Townsend, Davidson and Whitehead, 1988; Wilkinson, 1996). This report focuses on the little-researched issue of the factors that influence health-related behaviour in later life.

The proportion of older people in the population in Britain is increasing, especially those above age 75 (Central Statistical Office, 1996). There is considerable opportunity to improve the health-related behaviour of this section of the population (Ginn, Arber and Cooper, 1997), and thus to increase health expectancy (Bone *et al.*, 1995). As the proportion of older people in the population increases and older people consume an increasingly large proportion of health care, it is important to identify barriers faced by older people in adopting a healthy lifestyle. Our analysis focuses on men and women aged 55 and above, as a sizeable proportion of older people leave the labour market in their late 50s – particularly women – and reported ill-health increases for this age group (Bennett *et al.*, 1996).

There is a lack of detailed research evidence about the health-related behaviour of older people aged 55 and above, in terms of their lifestyles, smoking, drinking, diet and physical activity. In particular, less research has addressed class inequalities in health-related behaviour among older people than at other stages of the life course. This reflects both the tendency to see older people as a homogeneous group and the difficulties of measuring class for older people (Arber and Ginn, 1993). Class is sometimes considered problematic to measure for older people, who have generally left the labour market many years earlier. For older women, the conventional approach of classifying them by their husband's occupational class is of limited utility, because of the high proportion of older women who are widowed (see Table 1.2). However, research shows that class based on the older person's last main occupation reveals clear class gradients in health (Arber and Ginn, 1991, 1993; Arber and Cooper, 1999).

This report examines how an individual's lifestyle (diet, physical activity, smoking and drinking) is related to psychosocial factors, such as social support and family relationships, and material/structural variables, such as the older person's occupational class, income and housing circumstances. Since health status can affect lifestyle, our analyses take account of the older person's health where appropriate. A particular focus is how gender differentiates the pattern of these relationships, and to what extent these relationships differ for varying age groups among the older population and according to their marital status and living arrangements. We map class differences in lifestyles, health attitudes and involvement in health promotion strategies among older people.

A key issue is to what extent the factors associated with a healthy lifestyle are similar for different types of health-related behaviour. The report seeks to answer these questions and to identify the target groups of older people with particularly poor health and those who are most likely to engage in four types of health-damaging behaviour, namely smoking, high or excessive drinking, having a poor diet or taking a low level of physical exercise.

Datasets analysed

The research involves the analysis of four complementary national datasets.

1. The Health Survey for England, 1993 and 1994

The Health Survey for England (HSE) is an annual interview survey of adults living in about 10,000 private households in England (Colhoun and Prescott-Clarke, 1996). It contains extensive information on health behaviour, including detailed questions on diet, physical activity, smoking and drinking. In each survey, data are collected about psychosocial health, using the General Health Questionnaire (GHQ) and indicators of social support. This survey is analysed to provide detailed data on the health status and health risk factors (smoking, drinking, diet and physical activity) of five-year age groups of older people, and how these vary with their socioeconomic characteristics, marital status, living arrangements, psychosocial health and social support.

2. The General Household Survey, 1992–1994

The General Household Survey (GHS) is used to provide detailed information on the health status of older people, and their smoking and drinking behaviour (only asked in 1992 and 1994). The GHS interviews all adults aged 16 and over in about 10,000 private households in Britain each year, with a response rate of over 80% (Bennett *et al.*, 1996). The data analysed include the older person's income, housing tenure, car ownership, educational level, economic activity, occupational class and household circumstances, as well as their general health and whether they have any long-standing illness.

3. The Health Education and Monitoring Survey, 1995 and 1996

The Health Education and Monitoring Survey (HEMS) allows the analysis of health attitudes and beliefs about disease prevention of people aged 55–74, focusing on what factors influence underlying beliefs about health-promoting or health-damaging behaviour. The sample selection process was designed to yield a sample of approximately 5000 adults aged 16–74, one person in this age group selected for interview within each eligible household (Bridgwood *et al.*, 1996). A response rate of 76% was obtained. The analysis in this report has re-weighted the sample to take account of the differential probability of selection in different-sized households (i.e. respondents in larger households have a lower probability of selection) and the age–sex structure of the national population (see Bridgwood *et al.*, 1996). We use combined data from two years (1995 and 1996), yielding a sample of nearly 2800 people aged 55–74. The tables in this report are based on weighted data proportions and unweighted bases.

4. HEA Health and Lifestyles Survey, 1992

The HEA Health and Lifestyles Survey (HALS) was conducted by MORI in 1992 with a response rate of 75% (Health Education Authority, 1995). Our original intention was to use this survey to analyse the relationship between the lifestyle and health of different groups of older people, but the small number of older people interviewed (see Table 1.1) made this of limited value. This report only briefly refers to the HALS data, in Chapter 3 on smoking.

Demographic characteristics of older people aged 55+ in the four datasets

The research addresses the health-related behaviour and attitudes of people aged 55 and over. The analysis is based on over 18,000 people in three years of the General Household Survey (GHS), 1992–4; and represents about 11,000 men and women aged 55 and over in the 1993 and 1994 (combined) Health Survey for England (HSE), Table 1.1.

Table 1.1. Percentage of men and women aged 55+ in each dataset

	GHS 1992–4		HSE 1993–4		HEMS* 1995–6		HALS 1992	
	Men	Women	Men	Women	Men	Women	Men	Women
55–59	22.2	17.7	21.9	17.9	28.0	26.1	24.9	22.9
60–64	20.3	18.0	21.7	18.2	26.6	24.6	27.5	28.4
65–69	19.3	17.9	18.9	17.9	25.1	26.3	24.2	24.8
70–74	17.7	18.2	18.3	18.6	20.3	23.0	23.4	23.9
75–79	10.3	12.3	10.0	12.6				
80+	10.2	15.9	9.2	14.7				
Total (%)	100.0	100.0	100.0	100.0	100.0	100.0	100.0	100.0
N =	8280	10327	4771	6055	1265	1599	462	585

* HEMS proportions are weighted

The Health Education and Monitoring Survey (HEMS) and HEA Health and Lifestyles Survey (HALS) are smaller national datasets which did not include interviews with people aged 75 and over. Our analysis is based on about 2800 men and women aged 55–74 in the 1994 and 1995 (combined) HEMS and only 1000 people aged 55–74 in HEA HALS. The relatively small sample size of HALS meant that it was difficult to produce reliable analyses of different age groups of older people, therefore we have concentrated on the analysis of the other three datasets in this report.

The proportion of people in these four datasets is shown in Table 1.1 in 5-year-age groups from age 55 upwards. The higher mortality rate of older men than women can be seen from the percentages in each five-year age group in the GHS and HSE. A larger proportion of women than men are in age groups above 75, for example 16% of women are over 80 in the GHS compared to 10% of men.

Marital status is a key factor affecting the lives and living arrangements of older people and a main aim of this report is to understand how the interaction of marital status and gender influences older people's health-related behaviour. The likelihood of being widowed varies for older men and women and according to age group.

Table 1.2 shows that 77% of all men over age 55 are married compared with 52% of all women in the GHS. There is less gender difference in marital status among the 55–64 age group, but as age increases the gender difference becomes more pronounced. Over age 75, 63% of men are married compared with under a quarter of women, whereas nearly two-thirds of women (64%) are widowed compared with 30% of men. There are similar differences in marital status by age for men and women in the HSE (Table 1.3), and similarly the

Table 1.2. Marital status by age and sex: General Household Survey, 1992–4

	55–64		65–74		75+		All 55+	
	Men	**Women**	**Men**	**Women**	**Men**	**Women**	**Men**	**Women**
Married	82.5	73.6	77.5	52.9	62.8	24.6	76.6	52.3
Single	7.4	4.8	6.7	6.4	5.3	8.7	6.7	6.5
Widowed	4.0	14.1	11.7	35.8	30.0	64.0	12.2	36.0
Divorced	6.1	7.5	4.1	4.8	1.9	2.7	4.5	5.2
Total (%)	100.0	100.0	100.0	100.0	100.0	100.0	100.0	100.0
N =	3520	3684	3060	3726	1697	2915	8277	10325

Table 1.3. Marital status by age and sex: Health Survey for England, 1993–4

	55–64		65–74		75+		All 55+	
	Men	**Women**	**Men**	**Women**	**Men**	**Women**	**Men**	**Women**
Married	82.7	72.9	76.1	53.9	64.4	23.0	76.7	52.4
Single	6.4	3.7	6.6	6.4	5.3	8.3	6.3	5.9
Widowed	4.0	14.3	12.4	34.5	27.4	66.2	11.6	35.8
Divorced	6.8	9.1	5.0	5.2	2.8	2.5	5.4	5.9
Total (%)	100.0	100.0	100.0	100.0	100.0	100.0	100.0	100.0
N =	2078	2190	1772	2210	916	1653	4766	6053

Table 1.4. Marital status by age and sex: Health Education and Monitoring Survey, 1995–6

	55–64		65–74		All 55–74	
	Men	**Women**	**Men**	**Women**	**Men**	**Women**
Married	84.0	73.9	78.9	57.6	81.7	65.9
Single	5.7	3.9	6.0	5.7	5.8	4.8
Widowed	3.4	13.8	10.8	31.9	6.7	22.7
Divorced	6.9	8.3	4.4	4.8	5.8	6.6
Total (%)	100.0	100.0	100.0	100.0	100.0	100.0
N =	643	621	746	853	1264	1599

HEMS data show a greater proportion of men than women aged between 55 and 74 years are currently married (Table 1.4).

It is notable that only a relatively small proportion of older people are divorced or separated, and that this proportion decreases with advancing age, reflecting cohort differences in the propensity to divorce. However, the proportion who are divorced is higher for women in each age group, reflecting the greater likelihood of divorced men than women remarrying. The lifestyle of cohabitees may differ from that of the married. In some analyses, we therefore analyse cohabiting individuals separately from the married. However, because the numbers are very small, (under one per cent of men and women (n = 83) aged over 55 are cohabiting in the HSE), results must be treated with caution. Similarly, the numbers who are divorced or separated (as age advances) represent numerically small subgroups, and therefore the findings from these analyses may be unreliable.

Structure of report

Good health is essential if older people are to continue to contribute to society and to maintain a good quality of life. Health is the key concern of older people and the main determinant of their life satisfaction (Arber and Ginn, 1991; Sidell, 1995). Enabling older people to live healthy independent lives and remain in their own homes as long as possible benefits not only older people but society as a whole. Chapter 2 examines to what extent older people themselves have negative and fatalistic attitudes towards health, and what factors influence having fatalistic attitudes.

Chapter 3 examines smoking among older people, primarily using the GHS for 1992 and 1994 to analyse how smoking differs according to age, gender, marital status, living arrangements and socioeconomic characteristics, such as occupational class and housing tenure. This is supplemented where appropriate by additional analyses from the HSE and HALS.

Chapter 4 analyses levels of drinking among older men and women. Two sets of analyses are presented: first, for high drinking, that is above the recommended thresholds of 21 units per week for men and 14 units per week for women. Since there is controversy over whether these high levels represent behaviour which is damaging to health, our analyses have also been conducted for those defined as drinking 'excessively', that is 51 or more units per week for men and 36 or more units per week for women. Such 'excessive' drinking levels are likely to be health-damaging. Comparable analyses of drinking behaviour are conducted using the GHS for 1992 and 1994, as for smoking in Chapter 3, allowing a comparison of whether similar factors are associated with smoking and with high or excessive drinking.

Chapter 5 provides a detailed analysis of a range of physical activities undertaken by older people, focusing on how these vary between older men and women with advancing age and by marital status, using the HSE. A summary measure of physical activity is used which identifies those who engaged in little or no activity over the previous four weeks, defined here as 'sedentary'. Logistic regression is used to examine to what extent a range of social and economic factors are associated with a 'sedentary' lifestyle.

Chapter 6 analyses two health-related behaviours: smoking and diet, in a comparable set of analyses using the HSE. This chapter compares the extent to which these two health behaviours are affected by structural or material factors, such as occupational class, education, income and housing, compared with the older person's psychosocial health (measured by the General Health Questionnaire – GHQ), level of social support and living arrangements.

Chapter 7 draws conclusions about, first, the ways in which age, gender and health status are associated with health-related behaviour, second, the effects of marital status and living arrangements and the ways in which these affect the health behaviour of older men and women in different ways, and third, it highlights the importance of advantaged material circumstances in promoting good health behaviour, whereas disadvantaged circumstances are associated with health-damaging behaviour. The chapter also identifies the extent to which the same factors are associated with each of the four health-damaging behaviours: smoking, excessive drinking, a lack of physical activity and a poor diet, and highlights where there are differences between health behaviours. The final chapter also makes recommendations for future research.

2 Attitudes of older people concerning health

Introduction

This chapter uses data from the Health Education and Monitoring Survey (HEMS) to examine the attitudes of older people aged 55–74 years towards maintaining good health. We focus on the socioeconomic characteristics of those who display a 'fatalistic' attitude towards health, as measured by agreeing with the statement 'generally health is a matter of luck'. The tendency to view external factors, such as luck, as having a major influence on health reflects a reduced sense of personal control over determining good health. This may have implications for health behaviour and the perception of health promotion messages.

Qualitative research in this area has focused on lay definitions of health based on the in-depth study of small, localised samples or particular social groups (e.g. Pill and Stott, 1982, 1985; Davison, Frankel and Davey Smith, 1992) and has rarely considered older age groups in any detail. Whilst qualitative work is valuable, focusing on the individual should not detract from socioeconomic factors which may constrain or promote attitudes of control and responsibility for health (Becker, 1986). This is particularly important for older men and women who may experience changes in their socioeconomic circumstances associated with retirement and widowhood. Ageing and later life is often characterised as a time of increasing infirmity and dependency on others, which may also influence attitudes relating to personal control (Rodin, 1986).

There is a need to examine fatalistic attitudes about health within a wider perspective which acknowledges the heterogeneity of older age groups in terms of their socioeconomic position and health status. The social patterning of attitudes has clear implications for health promotion in this age group, as it may indicate the propensity or ability of older people to adopt a healthier lifestyle (Downie, Fyfe and Tannahill, 1992).

Fatalism and health

Individuals of all ages are increasingly encouraged to take personal responsibility for maintaining good health by adopting 'healthy lifestyle' behaviours, such as eating a balanced diet, taking regular exercise and the cessation of smoking. These health behaviours are viewed as being within the individual's self-control, and can be regulated to limit the risks of morbidity and mortality (Davison, Frankel and Davey Smith, 1992). Indeed, the emphasis given to these 'rational' behaviour choices has led to the conceptualisation of good health as being an actively pursued goal, a symbol of self-control and willpower (Crawford, 1984; Brownell, 1991).

Fatalism, or the belief that good health is primarily influenced by external forces outside of personal control, has been suggested as a factor underlying the apparent reluctance of some individuals to modify their health behaviour (Davison, Frankel and Davey Smith, 1992). Psychologists have extensively used 'locus of control' attitude scales to classify individuals into opposing 'internal' or 'external' groups based on their beliefs about the relative importance of their own actions and external influences, such as luck, chance and powerful others (Wallston, Wallston and Derellis, 1978). Externals or 'fatalists' are highlighted as those most likely to resist health education and behavioural change; the implicit assumption being that they lack responsibility and knowledge about their health, which must be rectified (Crawford, 1977, 1984).

Dean (1989) suggests that attitudes towards health are gendered, arising from differences in the socialisation of men and women. However, in a Danish study based on approximately 450 men and women aged 45+, there was no gender difference in perceived control of health, using the locus of control scale.

Qualitative research suggests that attitudes towards preserving good health are far more complex than the locus of control dichotomy allows. Pill and Stott (1985) devised a more flexible 'salience of lifestyle' index based on interviews with lower working-class mothers aged 25–40 years living in Wales. The index was constructed from scored responses to five questions about illness causation and prevention, according to whether lifestyle factors, such as diet and hygiene, were referred to in the response. The results showed that even when a high salience was given to lifestyle factors, this did not exclude responses which related to external influences about which they felt they had no personal control. Interviews with adults living in South Wales have also found that references to luck, chance and fate are very common in everyday discourse about health, yet individuals may modify their behaviour in an attempt to manipulate their luck (Davison, Frankel and Davey Smith, 1992).

Individuals appear to have the capacity to hold complex attitudes about the factors promoting their health, suggesting that it is misleading to assume that all fatalists deny the positive consequences of health-promoting behaviour, or that those with a healthy lifestyle do not acknowledge the existence of forces beyond their control. An undue emphasis on personal control and responsibility *per se* largely ignores the extent to which that control may be compromised by other factors, such as age, health status, class-related social norms and socioeconomic position (Townsend, Davidson and Whitehead, 1988).

Age and fatalism

Qualitative work has shown that respondents regularly refer to their position in the life course to account for and justify their health attitudes and lifestyle at different life stages (Backett and Davison, 1995). A greater premium is placed on good health (as measured by a quality of life index) during youth than at any other life stage, even by older respondents (Busschbach, Hessing and De Charro, 1993). Ageing is often associated with an inevitable decline in health and lower expectations about the benefits of health-promoting behaviour, such as exercise (Clark, 1996).

In a qualitative study based on adults living in South Wales, Davison, Frankel and Davey Smith (1992) found that references to luck, fate and chance were greatest among older age groups, with 47% of those aged between 65 and 71 years believing these factors influenced their health compared with 23% in the 18–31 age group.

This apparent increase in fatalism with age has also been observed in quantitative studies. Mirowsky (1995) used US survey data to examine levels of perceived control among adults aged 18–90 years, based on their responses to eight general attitude questions which did not specifically relate to their health. The results showed high and stable levels of control for those up to 50 years of age, but a consistent decrease in perceived control with older age. Other studies report less consistent results on the relationship between control and age, with a review of the American literature estimating that approximately one-third of studies claim low levels of control exist among older age groups, one-third show higher levels of control and the remainder show no association (Lachman, 1986). There has been much less British research on perceived control using large-scale data, but Lewis *et al.* (1989) report a strong association between increasing age and fatalistic attitudes to health, based on a survey of approximately 4000 adults living in Cardiff.

Understanding fatalism among older age groups

Health status

One explanation for the observed increase in fatalistic attitudes with age is that the greater physical impairment and disability experienced by older age groups serves to reduce their sense of personal control and autonomy (Mirowsky, 1995; Rodin, 1986). The association between functional disability and age is well established, with the ability to perform everyday tasks, such as walking and bathing, decreasing in progressively older age groups, especially for older women (Arber and

Cooper, 1999; Arber and Ginn, 1991). Increasing infirmity and dependency on others for assistance may therefore contribute to fatalistic attitudes about health. These attitudes may be reinforced by negative expectations about the future or by experiencing the loss of friends and family (Rodin, 1986).

Socioeconomic status

The propensity to view health in fatalistic terms may also be influenced by socioeconomic position. Pill and Stott (1985) found that a higher level of education among working-class mothers was significantly associated with a high score on the salience of lifestyle index, with these women more likely to reject the idea that their health was mainly influenced by luck. Neither parental social class nor home ownership was associated with attitudes to health in this group of women. Davison, Frankel and Davey Smith (1992) found no difference in attitudes between manual and non-manual groups, based on the analysis of semi-structured interviews, although ideas relating to luck were often discussed in the context of their living environment, workplace and family. However, significant class variation has been reported for all age groups in response to the statement that health is 'generally a matter of luck', with the manual classes more likely to agree than those in non-manual occupations (Lewis *et al.*, 1989).

Health and health behaviour among older people is clearly associated with socioeconomic position, based on such measures as social class, income and housing (Ginn, Arber and Cooper, 1997). Lower socioeconomic groups are more likely to suffer from poor health and also to engage in health-damaging behaviour than those in higher socioeconomic groups (Ginn, Arber and Cooper, 1997). Differences exist in the material resources of older men and women, with older women particularly disadvantaged compared with men of the same age (Arber and Ginn, 1991).

When examining the influence of socioeconomic position on the attitudes of older age groups, educational level emerges as a significant factor in explaining the association between age and perceived control. Mirowsky (1995), in a US study, reports that low educational attainment decreases the general sense of control among those aged 50 and above, and that educational level influences control to a greater extent than functional disability. Previous employment status and marital status did not influence the sense of control. However, those with a low level of household income were less likely to feel in control than those with higher income. One reason why education may have a greater influence on control than occupational class is that it reflects long-term social status, including childhood background and status as a young adult, as well as current social status. For example, poorer lifetime living and working conditions may culminate in a lower sense of control in old age. Education may also have an important role in developing skills of resourcefulness which bolster an individual's sense of personal control (Mirowsky, 1995).

Aims

Our research examines the prevalence of fatalism in relation to older people's attitudes towards health, based on the statement 'generally health is a matter of luck' (see Appendix B). Older people are classified as 'fatalist' if they agree or strongly agree that 'health is a matter of luck', and the remainder are combined into a 'non-fatalist' group. Previous work has shown significant social variation in responses to this question (Lewis *et al.*, 1989), but it is important to note that this single questionnaire item does not provide a personalised measure of fatalism. It is also unlikely to measure different dimensions of a fatalistic attitude which may be captured using a multi-item scale. Fatalistic health attitudes will be examined for men and women in different age groups to establish whether fatalism increases with advancing age.

One explanation for higher fatalism among older people is the higher prevalence of disability; therefore we consider whether older people reporting chronic illness or disability – as measured by long-standing illness (LI) and limiting long-standing illness (LLI) – are more likely to be fatalistic about health. The relationship between chronic health status and fatalism will be examined separately for older men and women to assess the effect of gender differences in chronic illness and disability in later life.

It does not necessarily follow that all fatalists deny the importance of personal behaviour on health. We therefore compare the factors rated as being good for health by older fatalists and non-fatalists to establish whether any differences exist between these groups in their propensity to acknowledge lifestyle factors affecting health.

There has been little research on socioeconomic factors associated with the health attitudes of older adults; therefore we examine how their social class, marital status, income and educational level are related to fatalistic attitudes about health. By controlling for age, sex and health status, we investigate whether the observed increase in fatalism in later life can be attributed to the disadvantaged structural position of older men and women, their health status or chronological age.

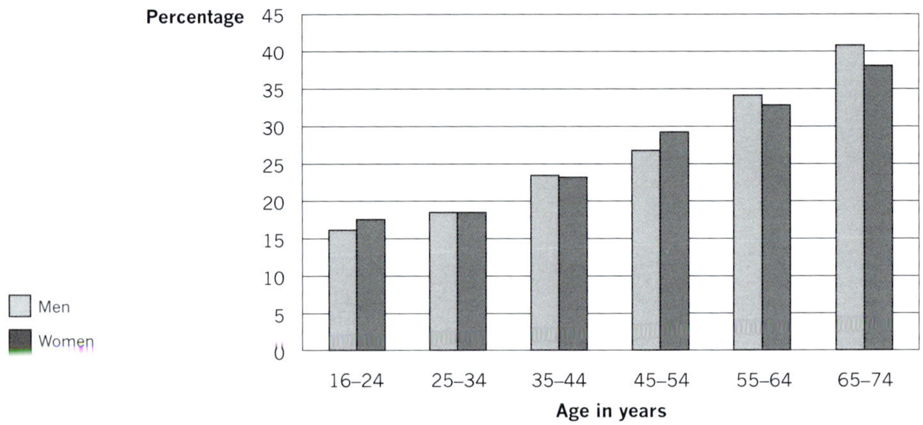

P < 0.001 for men and women

Source: Health Education and Monitoring Survey, 1995 and 1996

Figure 2.1. Percentage who agreed that health is a matter of luck by age and sex

Results

The percentage of men and women who agreed health is a matter of luck significantly increased with advancing age (Figure 2.1). Less than 20% of those under 35 years of age displayed a fatalistic attitude towards health, with comparable responses from men and women in these age groups. From age 35 upwards, fatalism increased progressively in each 10-year age group, with men more likely to agree with the statement than women in most age groups. For both sexes, fatalism increased by approximately 10% between the ages of 35–44 and 55–64, from 24% to 34% of respondents. Fatalistic health attitudes were most common among 65–74-year-olds, with 41% of men and 38% of women agreeing that luck influences health. This strong relationship between age and fatalism based on the 1995/6 HEMS survey supports previous research on fatalism and health (Davison, Frankel and Davey Smith, 1992; Lewis *et al.*, 1989) and age-related changes in the sense of control (Mirowsky, 1995).

When fatalism was examined in 5-year age groups for those aged 55+, a significant linear association between fatalism and age was still evident but was less clearly marked, especially for men (see Table 2.1). Approximately 35% of men and 32% of women aged 55–59 agreed that luck influences health, which increased to 42% for both sexes aged 70–74 years.

One previous explanation for the positive association between fatalism and age has been the higher morbidity of older age groups (Mirowsky, 1995). For example, an age-related increase in chronic ill

Table 2.1. Percentage of older men and women who agree that health is a matter of luck by age

	Age in years					
	55–59	**60–64**	**65–69**	**70–74**	**All 55–74**	***P* (Sig)**
Men	35	33	41	42	37	< 0.001
N =	(323)	(317)	(317)	(303)	(1260)	
Women	32	34	35	42	35	< 0.001
N =	(373)	(371)	(408)	(443)	(1595)	
All	34	33	38	42	36	< 0.001
N =	(696)	(688)	(725)	(746)	(2855)	

Source: Health Education and Monitoring Survey, 1995 and 1996

Table 2.2. Percentage reporting fatalistic health attitude by health status for men and women aged 55–74

	No chronic illness		**Limiting Illness**		**Limiting Long-standing Illness**		***P* (Sig)**
	%	***N***	**%**	***N***	**%**	***N***	
Men							
55–64	30	(303)	33	(125)	41	(212)	< 0.01
65–74	43	(274)	39	(141)	39	(205)	ns
All 55–74	36	(577)	36	(266)	40	(417)	< 0.01
Women							
55–64	35	(355)	27	(150)	34	(239)	ns
65–74	41	(370)	37	(170)	36	(311)	ns
All 55–74	33	(725)	32	(320)	35	(550)	ns

Source: Health Education and Monitoring Survey, 1995 and 1996

health and disability may account for the greater fatalism observed in the oldest age groups. However, Table 2.2 shows that limiting long-standing illness (LLI) was only significantly associated with increased fatalism for men aged 55–64, with 41% agreeing that health is a matter of luck, compared with 30% of those with no chronic illness. For men aged 65–74 and all women aged 55–74 years, health status and fatalism were not significantly associated. Overall, these results do not support the hypothesis that the increasing level of chronic ill health among older people contributes to the observed increase in fatalism with age.

Figure 2.2 (a–e) examines the factors rated as good for health by fatalists and non-fatalists to assess whether being fatalistic is consistent with

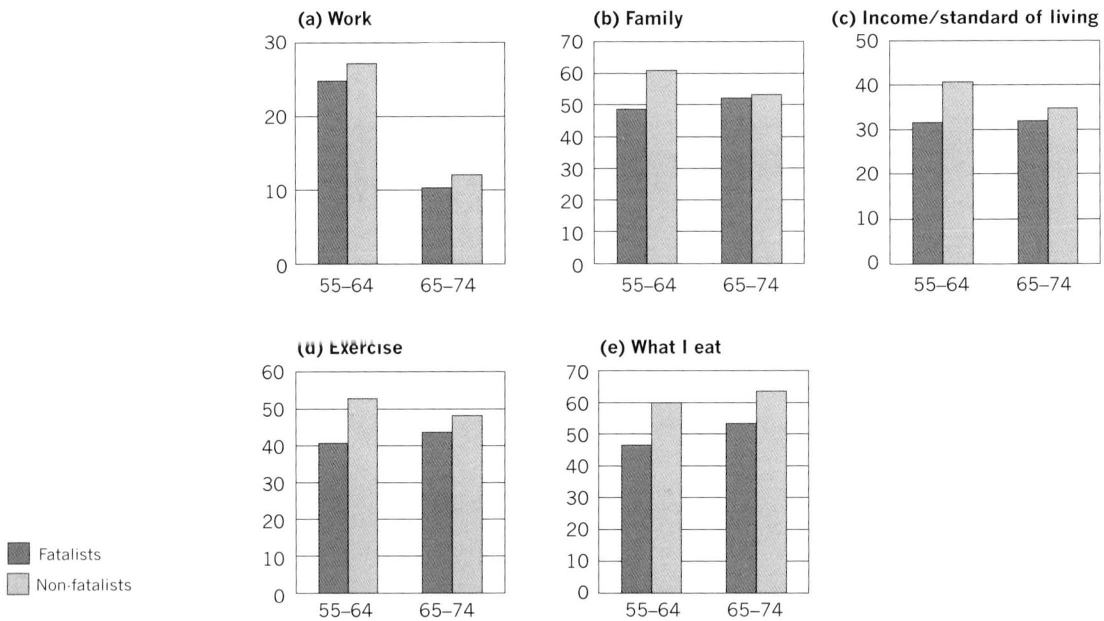

Source: Health Education and Monitoring Survey, 1995 and 1996

Fig. 2.2. Percentage viewing various factors as good for health by age and fatalism

placing a lower premium on individual health behaviour. Exercise and eating (Figure 2.2(d) and (e)) refer to health behaviours that individuals can alter, whereas work, family relationships and standard of living (Figure 2.2(a), (b) and (c)) are less susceptible to control by the individual.

Non-fatalists (who disagreed that luck influences health) were more likely to rate exercise and diet as being important for good health than fatalists. In both age groups of older people, non-fatalists were more likely to acknowledge the importance of exercise, compared with fatalists, especially in the 55–64 age group. Diet was rated as important for health by approximately 60% of non-fatalists, but this decreased to just over half of fatalists aged 65–74 and was below 50% for 55–64-year-old fatalists. Non-fatalists were also more likely to view income/ standard of living as being important for good health than fatalists, especially those aged 55–64, but family relationships were rated as highly likely to influence health by all respondents, regardless of their health attitude. Not surprisingly, the perceived importance of work for health decreased markedly with age for both groups, as individuals aged 65 and above are likely to have retired from paid work. The results in Figure 2.2 are consistent with a belief system in which fatalists attach a lower priority to the role of health behaviours in determining good health than non-fatalists. However, there is no consistent evidence

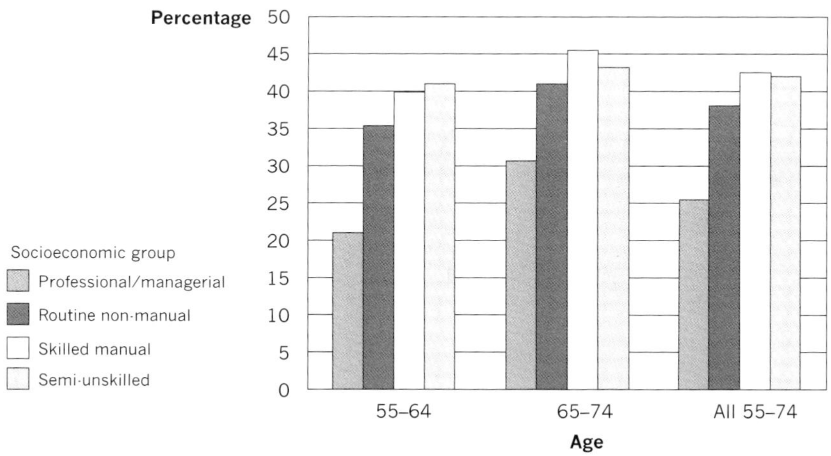

$P < 0.001$ for all age groups

Source: Health Education and Monitoring Survey, 1995 and 1996

Fig. 2.3. Percentage who agreed health is a matter of luck by age and socioeconomic group

of decline between 55–64 and 65–74 years in the propensity to rate the various sorts of health behaviour as good for health; in fact a greater proportion of both fatalists and non-fatalists aged 65+ rated diet as important for good health.

We now focus on the socioeconomic characteristics of those displaying a fatalistic attitude towards health to assess whether the material living conditions and social position of older men and women exerts an influence on this health attitude. Figure 2.3 shows a significant association between social class (as measured by socioeconomic group based on the older person's last main occupation – see Appendix A) and fatalism.

Older men and women who currently or last worked in semi- and unskilled occupations were more likely to agree that health is a matter of luck than those in professional and managerial occupations. Within the 55–64-year age group, over 40% of those in semi-skilled or unskilled occupations expressed a fatalistic attitude, which decreased to 35% for routine non-manual workers and was only 22% for the professional and managerial class. For older people aged 65–74 years, fatalism was greatest in the skilled manual class, with fatalistic attitudes towards health substantially lower for those in non-manual classes.

Fatalism was strongly associated with the educational qualifications of older men and women aged 55–64 and 65–74 years, as shown in Figure 2.4. For both age groups, those with no formal qualifications were substantially more likely to be fatalistic about health than those with a higher qualification. For all aged 55–74, there was a linear decrease in fatalistic attitudes as levels of formal education increased,

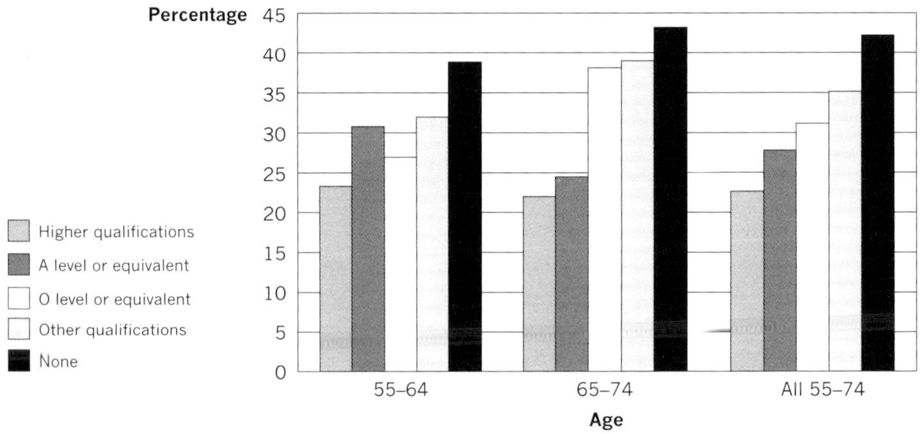

$P < 0.001$ for all age groups

Source: Health Education and Monitoring Survey, 1995 and 1996

Fig. 2.4. Percentage who agreed health is a matter of luck by age and highest educational qualification

with fatalism at approximately 41% among the unqualified, falling to 31% with O-level qualifications, 27% with A-levels and was lowest at 23% for the highly educated.

Multivariate analysis of fatalism for older men and women

Using logistic regression, it is possible to examine the association between a range of socioeconomic factors and fatalism after controlling for age and gender differences in the prevalence of this attitude. Using this method, we can determine the extent to which fatalism can be attributed to the social class or educational level of older age groups, and whether chronic ill-health is associated with greater fatalism for older men and women after controlling for these factors. The odds ratios for being fatalistic are first presented for all older people aged 55–74 (Table 2.3), and then separately for men and women (Table 2.4), in order to examine whether gender differences that exist in socioeconomic position and health status for this age group influence fatalistic attitudes for older men and women.

All aged 55–74

Model 1 (Table 2.3) includes age, sex and marital status. There was some increase in the odds ratio of being fatalistic with advancing age, but this was only statistically significant for the oldest age group of 70–74-year-olds. Older women appear to be less fatalistic than men, with their odds of being fatalistic reduced by 14% compared with men (the reference category), although this difference is not statistically

Table 2.3. Odds ratios for logistic regression of fatalism for all aged 55–74

	Model 1	Model 2	Model 3	Model 4
Age	ns	ns	ns	ns
55–59	1.00	1.00	1.00	1.00
60–64	0.92	0.88	0.89	0.89
65–69	1.21	1.14	1.16	1.16
70–74	1.38 **	1.26 *	1.29 *	1.30 *
Sex	ns	†	†	ns
Male	1.00	1.00	1.00	1.00
Female	0.86	0.81 **	0.85	0.85
Marital status	ns	ns	ns	ns
Married/cohabiting	1.00	1.00	1.00	1.00
Single	1.29	1.25	1.23	1.22
Widowed	1.03	0.95	0.95	0.95
Divorced/separated	0.90	0.90	0.87	0.86
Educational level		†††	††	††
Higher		1.00	1.00	1.00
A level or equivalent		1.36	1.25	1.27
O level or equivalent		1.58 ***	1.34 *	1.37 *
Other		1.81 ***	1.40 *	1.41 **
None		2.42 ***	1.72 ***	1.72 ***
Socioeconomic group			†††	†††
Professional/managerial			1.00	1.00
Routine non-manual			1.40 **	1.39 **
Skilled manual			1.72 ***	1.71 ***
Semi-/Unskilled			1.42 **	1.41 **
Housing tenure			ns	ns
Owner occupier			1.00	1.00
Local authority			1.20	1.18
Private renter			1.06	1.06
Chronic health status				ns
No chronic illness				1.00
Long-standing illness (LI)				0.83
Limiting long-standing illness (LLI)				1.04
Δ –2LLR	24.5	65.8	29.4	5.3
Δ df	7	4	5	2
N =	2048			

Statistical significance of variable in the model: † $P < 0.05$; †† $P < 0.01$; ††† $P < 0.001$.

Statistical significance of difference from reference category: * $P < 0.05$; ** $P < 0.01$; *** $P < 0.001$.

Source: Health Education and Monitoring Survey, 1995 and 1996

significant. There was some suggestion that older single people are more likely to be fatalistic relative to the married and previously married, but these gender and marital status differences were not statistically significant.

Adding educational level in Model 2 substantially improved the overall fit of the model by 65.8. There was a clear linear increase in the likelihood of being fatalistic about health as the level of education decreased, with the unqualified over twice as likely to view luck as a factor in health compared with those with higher qualifications. Including education in the model resulted in the gender difference observed in Model 1 becoming statistically significant, with older women being significantly less likely to be fatalistic than older men. However, once education was included in the model, the association between age and fatalism became somewhat weaker. This could reflect cohort differences in education, for example, if the average levels of education are lower among the oldest age groups compared with those in their late 50s and early 60s (Mirowsky, 1995).

Model 3 shows a statistically significant but non-linear social class gradient in the odds ratios of being fatalistic after controlling for the other factors in the model. The skilled manual class had their odds significantly increased by 72% relative to the professional and managerial group. Housing tenure did not make any significant contribution to the model. The gradient observed for education in Model 3 was slightly weakened when social class and housing were added to the model, but the odds of being fatalistic remained significantly higher for those with lower level or no qualifications relative to the reference category.

Having a LLI did not significantly increase the likelihood of holding fatalistic attitudes about health; the odds for those with LLI and LI were comparable with the reference category of no chronic illness (Model 4). Adding health status to the model did not alter the strong association between education and fatalism, and the skilled manual class also remained more likely to be fatalistic.

These results show that educational level is an important determinant of fatalism for those aged 55–74 years. This confirms previous US research on older people (Mirowsky, 1995) and is comparable to the findings from qualitative work on younger age groups (Pill, Peters and Robling, 1993). A higher level of education may positively relate to the acquisition of skills, such as problem-solving and self-reliance. These skills may foster an increased sense of personal control which extends to attitudes and beliefs about health.

Men and women aged 55–74

Table 2.4 (Model 1) examines differences between men and women in the factors associated with having a fatalistic health attitude. Men aged 65–74 and women in their early 70s were most likely to be fatalistic, but marital status did not influence attitudes about luck and health.

Table 2.4. Odds ratios for logistic regression of fatalism for men and women aged 55–74

	Men			Women		
	Model 1	Model 2	Model 3	Model 1	Model 2	Model 3
Age	ns	ns	ns	ns	ns	ns
55–59	1.00	1.00	1.00	1.00	1.00	1.00
60–64	0.86	0.84	0.80	1.01	0.92	0.95
65–69	1.40 *	1.29	1.30	1.05	1.02	1.05
70–74	1.41 *	1.27	1.27	1.36 *	1.25	1.33
Marital status	ns	ns	ns	ns	ns	ns
Married/cohabiting	1.00	1.00	1.00	1.00	1.00	1.00
Single	1.57	1.47	1.41	1.10	1.19	1.23
Widowed	1.24	1.16	1.16	0.94	0.89	0.87
Divorced/separated	1.13	1.06	1.02	0.71	0.78	0.76
Educational level		†††	ns		†††	†††
Higher		1.00	1.00		1.00	1.00
A level or equivalent		1.07	1.03		2.03 *	1.81
O level or equivalent		1.09	0.94		2.41 ***	2.08 ***
Other		1.72 ***	1.35		2.03 ***	1.59 *
None		1.73 ***	1.23		3.49 ***	2.53 ***
Socioeconomic group			††			†
Professional/managerial			1.00			1.00
Routine non-manual			1.55			1.36
Skilled manual			1.64 ***			1.85 **
Semi-/unskilled			1.14			1.56 *
Housing tenure			ns			ns
Owner occupier			1.00			1.00
Local authority			1.12			1.01
Private renter			1.31			1.06
Chronic health status			ns			†
No chronic illness			1.00			1.00
Long-standing illness (LI)			0.98			0.69
Limiting long-standing illness (LLI)			1.29			0.85
Δ –2LLR	21.9	22.3	26.4	8.4	56.0	18.4
Δ df	6	4	7	6	4	7
N=	926			1143		

Statistical significance of variable in the model: † $P < 0.05$; †† $P < 0.01$; ††† $P < 0.001$.

Statistical significance of difference from reference category: * $P < 0.05$; ** $P < 0.01$; *** $P < 0.001$.

Source: Health Education and Monitoring Survey, 1995 and 1996

Model 2 shows that a low level of education significantly increased the odds ratios of being fatalistic, improving the fit of the model by 56.0 for older women and 22.3 for older men (Model 2). Among women with no formal qualifications, the odds of agreeing that health is a matter of luck were over three times greater than for highly qualified women. The odds also increased for those with 'other' and A-level or O-level qualifications relative to the reference category of higher education. Unqualified older men had their odds of being fatalistic increased by 73% compared with the highly qualified, a difference which was much less than for women but was still statistically significant.

Class was significantly associated with fatalism for men and women (Model 3). Men in the skilled manual class and women in the manual classes were significantly more likely to be fatalistic relative to the reference category of professional and managerial workers. Men previously employed in routine non-manual occupations also had a higher odds ratio of being fatalistic, but this was not statistically significant. Adding socioeconomic group to the model resulted in education becoming non-significant for older men, but not for older women. For women, a low level of education remained strongly associated with fatalistic health attitudes.

The odds ratios of fatalism increased for men reporting a LLI; however, this odds ratio was not significantly different from men with no chronic illness after controlling for age and socioeconomic position (Model 3). There was a significant inverse relationship between health status and fatalism for older women; fatalistic attitudes were less likely among women with a LI or LLI illness than for women with no chronic illness. This is an important finding given that levels of functional disability and chronic ill-health are greater among older women than older men.

Discussion and conclusions

Our results confirm that fatalistic attitudes about health are clearly differentiated by age, as fatalism increased between mid-adulthood and later life. However, within older age groups, the relationship between age and fatalism was relatively modest, especially after controlling for socioeconomic and gender differences. Our results highlight the heterogeneity of older age groups and the importance of examining gender and socioeconomic influences on health attitudes.

We found no strong evidence that chronic illness among older people contributes to greater fatalistic attitudes towards health. LLI was only significantly associated with fatalism for men aged 55–64 and our results suggested that fatalism was lower for women with reported chronic health problems than for those with no chronic illness.

Those who rejected luck as a factor in health were more likely than fatalists to acknowledge lifestyle factors, such as diet and exercise, as important for maintaining good health. Acknowledging the importance of individual health behaviour suggests a more autonomous view of good health as being within personal control, and in this respect having a fatalistic health attitude may reduce the likelihood of older adults engaging in preventive health behaviour.

The most important factor in explaining the health attitudes of older people was their educational level. The highly educated were least likely to be fatalistic, especially women. Educational level may have an important role in the development of life skills and resourcefulness, especially for women. Possessing these skills may encourage a greater sense of individual responsibility and control which extends to attitudes about health and engaging in health behaviour.

The results from our analysis suggest that socioeconomic resources do influence the tendency to be fatalistic about health; a low social class position was associated with greater fatalism, particularly for older men, whereas low education had a greater influence on fatalism among older women. It is important to consider how earlier occupational roles and associated material resources, as well as cultural resources, such as education, may constrain or promote individual lifestyle choices for men and women.

3 How class and living circumstances relate to smoking behaviour among older people

Introduction

This chapter examines the effect of class and living circumstances on cigarette smoking among those aged 55 and above, using data from three British surveys: the GHS, the HSE and the HEA HALS. We consider the smoking behaviour of older men and women according to their socioeconomic position, current living circumstances and health status. Daily cigarette consumption is also examined in order to highlight the socioeconomic characteristics of those most likely to be 'heavy smokers'. As our analysis is concerned with the current smoking behaviour of older people, we do not distinguish between ex-smokers and those who have never smoked.

Smoking has been cited as the main cause of lung cancer, with an estimated one-fifth of deaths in the UK attributable to tobacco (Health Education Authority, 1996). A key concern of government policy is to reduce the morbidity and mortality associated with smoking (Department of Health, 1998, 1996). However, older people tend to be neglected by anti-smoking initiatives, although this age group represent the fastest growing segment of the population (White, 1997) and smoking remains the leading cause of chronic illness and premature death among older adults (Greengross *et al.*, 1997; Orleans *et al.*, 1991). Figures from the GHS show that although the prevalence of smoking has decreased over the last 20 years for all age groups, the rate of this decline was much lower among older people aged 60 and above (Bennett *et al.*, 1996).

Despite the overall decrease in cigarette smoking over recent years, it is increasingly concentrated among those living in the most disadvantaged socioeconomic circumstances (Dawes and Goddard, 1997; Bennett *et al.*, 1996; Bridgwood *et al.*, 1996; Health Education Authority, 1995; Marsh and McKay, 1994; Townsend, 1992). Individuals in the lowest social groups are more likely to smoke than those in the higher social groups, based on both individual and household measures of social class. However, the extent of this social variation is not examined in any detail for older age groups, and it is unclear how social class and deprived living conditions are associated with smoking behaviour in later life.

There is evidence that marital status may influence smoking behaviour, with the loss of a partner through death or divorce associated with smoking and greater cigarette consumption for men and women.

However, these results are often presented for all adults aged 16+, with the widowed and divorced being combined into one category (Bennett *et al.*, 1996; Department of Health, 1996; Bridgwood *et al.*, 1995). This is potentially misleading in two respects. First, both marital status and smoking are known to be heavily age-dependent, and second, important differences may exist between divorced and widowed men and women in their socioeconomic circumstances, health and health-related behaviour. By using large-scale data, our study examines smoking among the over-55s in detail according to their age, marital status and living arrangements, differentiating between the divorced and widowed and those living alone and with other people.

Age-related trends in cigarette smoking

GHS data show a consistent decrease in cigarette smoking for all age groups over the last two decades (Wald and Nicolaides-Bouman, 1991; Bennett *et al.*, 1996; Osler, 1993) from 51% of men and 41% of women in 1974 to around one-quarter of all adults in 1994 (Bennett *et al.*, 1996). Smoking is most prevalent in the 20–24-year age group at around 40% and then consistently decreases with age to 18% among older adults aged 60 and above (Bennett *et al.*, 1996). Up to the age of 60, the average number of cigarettes smoked per day increases with age, with older smokers over 60 years having a similar level of cigarette consumption to smokers in their twenties (Bennett *et al.*, 1996).

Men are more likely to smoke than women, but this gender difference has narrowed over time, particularly for older age groups. In 1974, men aged 60+ were three times more likely to smoke than women of the same age (Bennett *et al.*, 1996), but data from the 1996 Omnibus survey show higher smoking among older women aged 55–64 and 65–74 years than for older men, with comparable smoking for both sexes aged 75+ at 10% (Dawes and Goddard, 1997).

Figure 3.1 confirms this age-related decrease in cigarette smoking based on two years of data from the GHS. The proportion of non-smokers increased with advancing age for both sexes, from approximately 66% of men and women aged 16–24 years to around three-quarters of 55–64-year-olds and was over 90% among the oldest age group, aged 85+. Women were slightly more likely to smoke than men up to the age of 45 years, and there was no gender difference in smoking for those aged between 45 and 74 years. Only within the oldest age groups (75+ years) were men more likely to smoke than women.

Clear gender differences were found in cigarette consumption, with

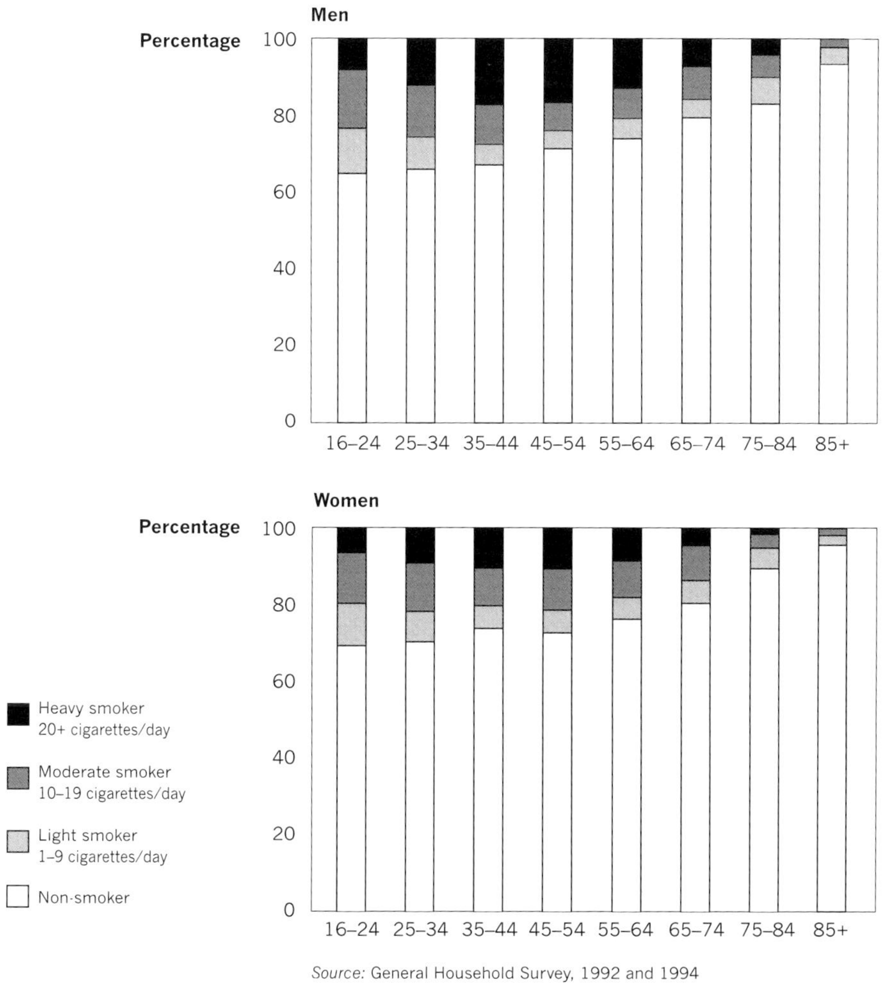

Fig. 3.1. Smoking status of men and women by age group, aged 16+

men more likely to be heavy smokers (smoking 20+ cigarettes per day) than women in each age group. For both sexes, heavy smoking increased during early adulthood and was greatest among those aged between 35 and 54. From 55 upwards, heavy smoking consistently decreased with age, with no heavy smoking among older men and women aged 85+.

The decline in smoking and high cigarette consumption with age is likely to be for two main reasons, first, because of the higher mortality rate of smokers. Survivors are disproportionately non-smokers, an effect which increases with advancing age. Second, because of ill-health those who smoke are likely to be advised by their doctors to give up smoking. Our results from the HEA HALS show that 14% of men and 30% of women aged between 55 and 74 years who used to be regular smokers gave up smoking because of health problems or advice from their doctor. Analysis of the Health Survey for England (Colhoun and Prescott-Clarke, 1996) confirms that a general decline in smoking between 1991 and 1994 among adults aged 65 and above can be attributed to smoking cessation during this period.

The narrowing gender difference in smoking may reflect cohort differences in lifetime smoking behaviour. Women have increasingly taken up smoking since the Second World War (Wald and Nicolaides-Bouman, 1991), whereas women in their 70s and 80s belong to a generation of women who were unlikely to smoke during adulthood. The number of older women who have never smoked decreased from 63% in 1974 to 54% in 1994, unlike other age groups, where there has been an increase in non-smokers over this period (Bennett *et al.*, 1996).

Gender differences in smoking in later life thus reflect distinct gendered processes relating to cohort changes in smoking behaviour, as well as the relationship between smoking and ill health, and smoking and mortality. Cross-sectional data, such as the GHS, do not allow us to isolate the varying contributions of these three factors to the decline in smoking with increasing age.

Socioeconomic status and smoking behaviour

Strong social class variation in smoking has been reported for all adults aged 16 and above (Bennett *et al.*, 1996; Bridgwood *et al.*, 1996; Health Education Authority, 1995; Wald and Nicolaides-Bouman, 1991). In 1996, 12% of professional men and 19% of professional women smoked, compared with 35% of women and 38% of men in unskilled manual occupations (Dawes and Goddard, 1997).

The finding that smoking is greatest among disadvantaged social groups has been clearly demonstrated for lone parents (Dorsett and Marsh, 1998; Marsh and Matheson, 1983), women of low socio-economic status (Graham, 1993) and those who do not own their own homes (Health Education Authority, 1995; Marsh and McKay, 1994). A Policy Studies Institute survey in 1994 based on over 2000 low-income families reported that smoking prevalence increased among those living on low income, with no educational qualifications, living in council housing and from manual occupations (Marsh and McKay, 1994). The likelihood of giving up smoking was greater among the more affluent social groups, with three-quarters of families living on Income Support still smoking. This sample was based on low-income families receiving child benefit, hence older people are likely to be under-represented. Little is known about the prevalence of smoking among older people in relation to their material living circumstances. Changes in socioeconomic circumstances are likely to occur in later life, for example, as older people leave the labour market and experience changes in their income or marital status. Our study uses several indicators of social disadvantage to analyse how the smoking behaviour of older men and women is associated with their social class, income and housing.

Evidence suggests that marital dissolution is associated with greater smoking prevalence and cigarette consumption among adults aged 16 and above (Bennett *et al.*, 1996; Bridgwood *et al.*, 1996; Department of Health, 1996), especially for men. Figures from the 1994 GHS show 18% of widowed and divorced men smoke heavily compared with around one-tenth of single and married men, but that there is little difference in the smoking behaviour of adult women according to their marital status (Bennett *et al.*, 1996).

Using national survey data from America, Umberson (1992) found that divorce was associated with cigarette smoking for men and women after controlling for age-related differences in this health behaviour. Widowhood was also associated with smoking, but only for men. These results are confirmed by Wyke and Ford (1992) who found that 55-year-olds who were no longer married (the widowed and divorced combined) were less likely to be non-smokers or ex-smokers than the married or single. However, there was some evidence to suggest that the previously married and single men have less material resources than their married counterparts, as measured by car ownership. The loss of a spouse has also been associated with greater psychological distress and lower perceived levels of social support (Umberson, 1992; Wyke and Ford, 1992).

Marriage may therefore be beneficial to individuals in terms of available socioeconomic resources and social support, with some evidence that men benefit from a more 'orderly' lifestyle within marriage (Umberson, 1987) and from having their health-related behaviour monitored by their spouse (Umberson, 1992). When studying the smoking behaviour of older people it is therefore important to take into account any underlying differences in the socioeconomic position of widowed, divorced, single and married men and women.

Aims

Using large-scale survey data we examine the association between socioeconomic characteristics and smoking behaviour for men and women aged 55 and above. We assess the social determinants of whether or not an individual smokes as well as any social variation in cigarette consumption, based on measures of social class, income and housing tenure (see Appendix A). Our measure of housing tenure divides those living in owner occupier, privately rented and local authority/housing association accommodation, and distinguishes between owner occupiers and local authority tenants who have been resident for five years or more or for less than five years (owing to the small numbers of older people in privately rented accommodation, it was not possible to make this distinction). This will highlight those who have moved house in recent years, possibly moving in with relatives owing to increasing infirmity. Any change in living environment is likely to be disruptive and stressful and may have consequences for health behaviour. Our study investigates how social class and living conditions, which are strongly associated with smoking behaviour in the general adult population, influence smoking among older age groups of men and women.

A particular concern is to extend and clarify previous work which has suggested that marital status is associated with smoking behaviour. We analyse the current living arrangements of older people in some detail to investigate whether marital dissolution influences smoking for this age group. For widowed and never-married older people, we distinguish between those living alone and those living with others (the small numbers of divorced/separated older men and women meant that it was not possible to distinguish their living arrangements in this way). This may highlight any differences that exist between these groups in terms of potential social support and attempts by others to monitor their health behaviour.

Using multivariate logistic regression, our analysis controls for a range of socioeconomic factors to determine their relative influence on smoking. It is possible to examine the extent to which non-married older men and women are disadvantaged in terms of their living conditions relative to the married, which may have implications for their smoking behaviour.

Age differences in smoking and cigarette consumption

Figure 3.2 shows the proportion of men and women who smoked by five-year age groups from age 55 upwards. There was a substantial decline in smoking with increasing age for both sexes. This was especially marked for women, with only 6% aged 80+ currently smoking compared with 23% in their late 60s and 27% aged 55–59 years. There was little gender difference in cigarette smoking for men and

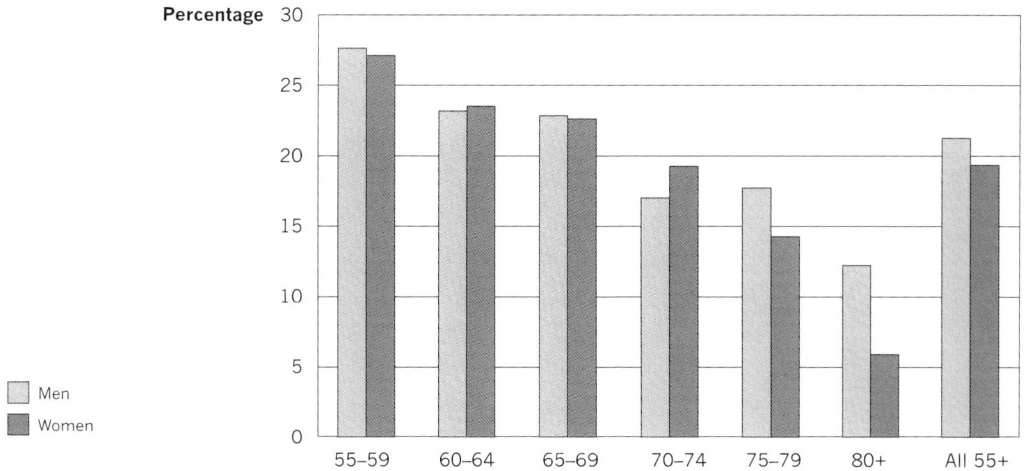

Source: General Household Survey, 1992 and 1994

Fig. 3.2. Percentage currently smoking cigarettes by age and sex, aged 55+

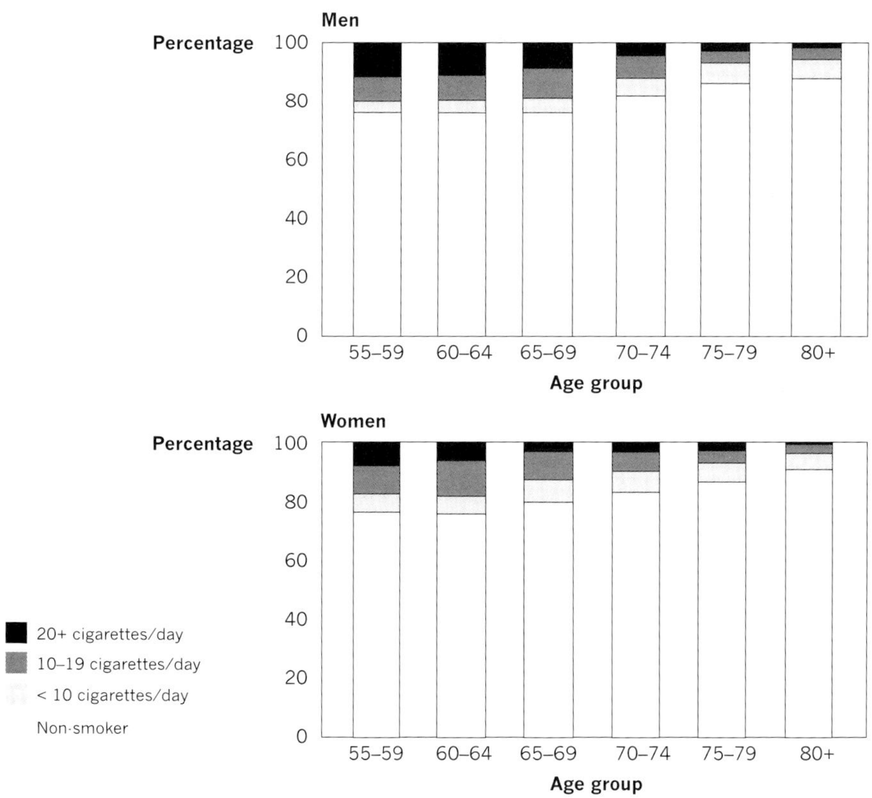

Source: Health Survey for England, 1993 and 1994

Fig. 3.3. Smoking status of men and women by age group, aged 55+

women in their late 50s and 60s, but a greater proportion of women in the 70–74-year age group were current smokers than men. Over the age of 75 years, men were more likely to smoke than women, with twice as many men than women smoking at age 80 and above. These results confirm that the gender difference in smoking behaviour is narrowing, and suggests that younger generations of women are more likely to smoke than older women in their late 70s or above.

Figure 3.3 shows the percentage of older men and women who were non-smokers as well as the cigarette consumption of current smokers, based on two years of data from the HSE. Similar to the GHS results shown in Figure 3.2, the proportion of non-smokers increased with age for older men and women, and within age groups the gender differences in smoking were small. Heavy smoking decreased with age for both sexes, but older men were more likely to smoke 20+ cigarettes a day than older women in each age group.

Socioeconomic differences in smoking and cigarette consumption

When smoking behaviour was examined by socioeconomic group, the results showed that older men in manual social classes have higher rates of smoking than professional/managerial men (Figure 3.4). Over twice as many men aged 55–64 years in the semi- and unskilled class smoked compared with professional and managerial men of the same age. Clear social class gradients in smoking were observed in all age groups up to age 75+, despite the effects of selective survival relating to class and smoking behaviour.

For older women, there was a clear class difference in smoking for those aged 55–64 years, with approximately 33% of women in manual occupations smoking compared with 20% of those in the non-manual social classes. With increasing age, the class differences in smoking became more inconsistent, with the lowest levels of smoking observed for skilled manual class among women aged 75 and above. This is likely to reflect cohort differences in smoking; the smaller proportion of older women who smoke are less class divided than for men.

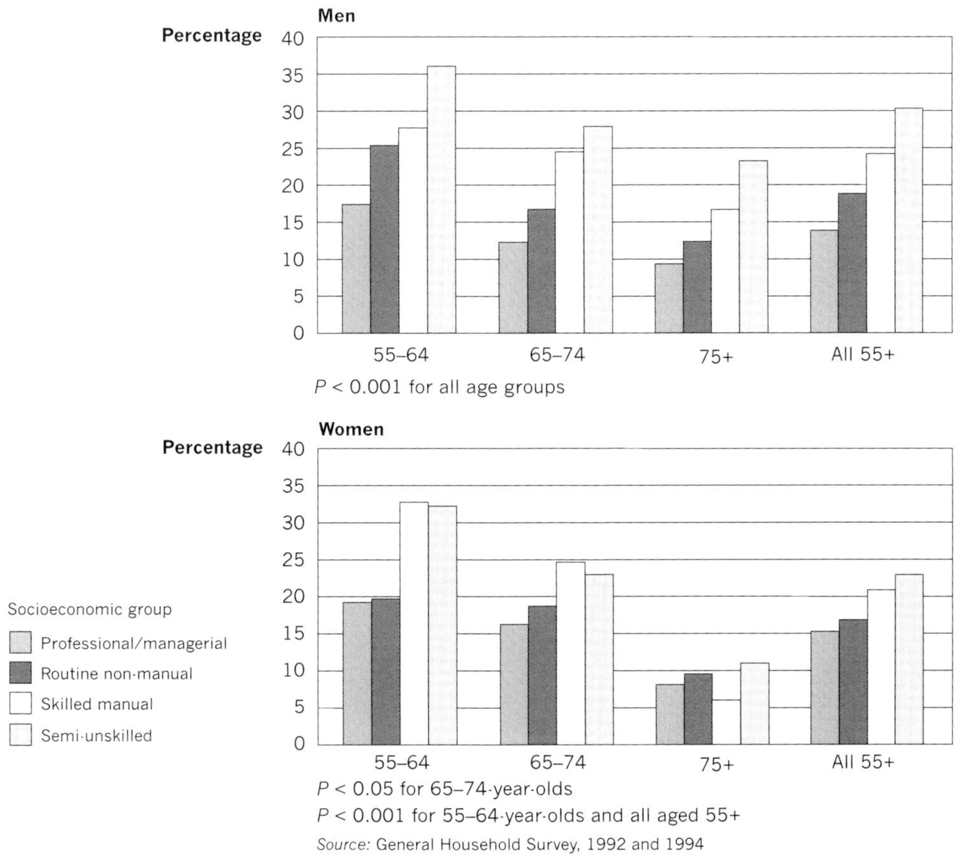

Fig. 3.4. Percentage of current cigarette smokers by age and socioeconomic group

Figure 3.5 shows an inverse association between smoking and income for older men; the proportion of non-smokers consistently decreased as household income decreased (household income is equivalised to take into account the number of adults living in the household – see Appendix A). Men in the lowest 20% of household income were most likely to be current smokers and to smoke heavily, with 11% in this group smoking 20 or more cigarettes a day compared with 8% in the highest income group. For women, the relationship between income and cigarette consumption was more curved, with women in the middle and lowest quintiles of the income distribution slightly more likely to smoke. For both sexes, a higher proportion of light smokers (1–9 cigarettes per day) were found in the lowest income groups, which could reflect the financial implications of a heavy smoking habit among this group.

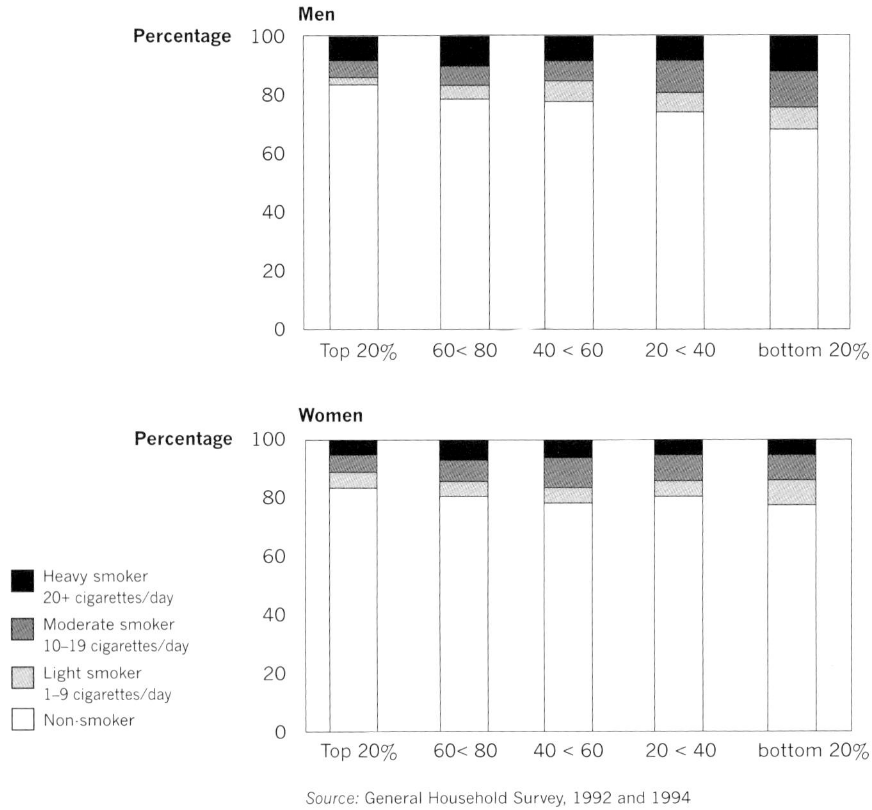

Fig. 3.5. Smoking status of men and women by equivalised household income, aged 55+

The living arrangements of older people were significantly associated with their smoking behaviour (Figure 3.6). For all men aged 55 and above, smoking was substantially higher among the divorced/ separated, with 40% of smokers in this group compared with the lowest smoking of 19% for married men. Single men living alone also had high levels of smoking (27%), whilst being widowed and living with others was associated with greater smoking for both sexes. Similar to older men, women who were divorced or separated had the highest levels of smoking at 26%, and comparable levels of smoking were observed between married men and women at 18%. However, unlike older men, the lowest levels of smoking were found for single women, with only one-tenth of those living with others currently smoking. These differences are consistent with the hypothesis that marriage promotes healthier behaviours, particularly for men, and that divorce is associated with more health-damaging smoking behaviour for older men and women.

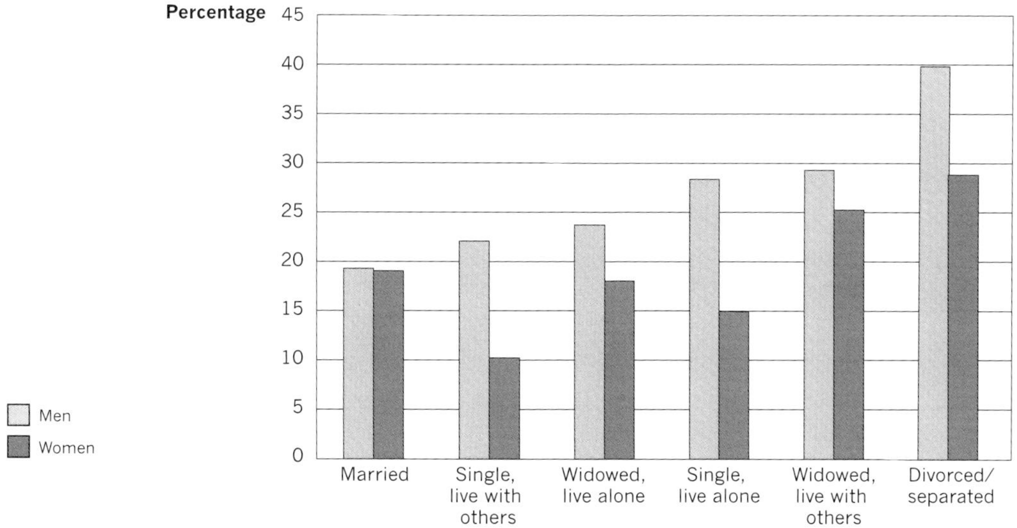

P < 0.01 for men and women

Source: General Household Survey, 1992 and 1994

Fig. 3.6. Percentage of men and women aged 55+ currently smoking cigarettes by living arrangements

When these marital status differences were examined according to age (Figure 3.7) the results confirmed that divorced men aged 65 and above are much more likely to smoke than widowed, single or married men. This was particularly marked among men aged 75+, where 32% of divorced men smoked compared with 16% of widowed men and 14% of married men. For younger men aged 55–64 years, smoking was slightly higher among the widowed, but smoking remained high among the divorced compared with married and single men. Married men below the age of 75 years were least likely to smoke. For women under the age of 75 years, smoking was greatest among the divorced/ separated and widowed. Approximately 34% of widowed and divorced women smoked at age 55–64 years, which fell to 23% among the married and 21% for single women. Levels of smoking were much lower for all women in the oldest age group, but divorced/separated women continued to have levels of smoking that were twice as great as the married.

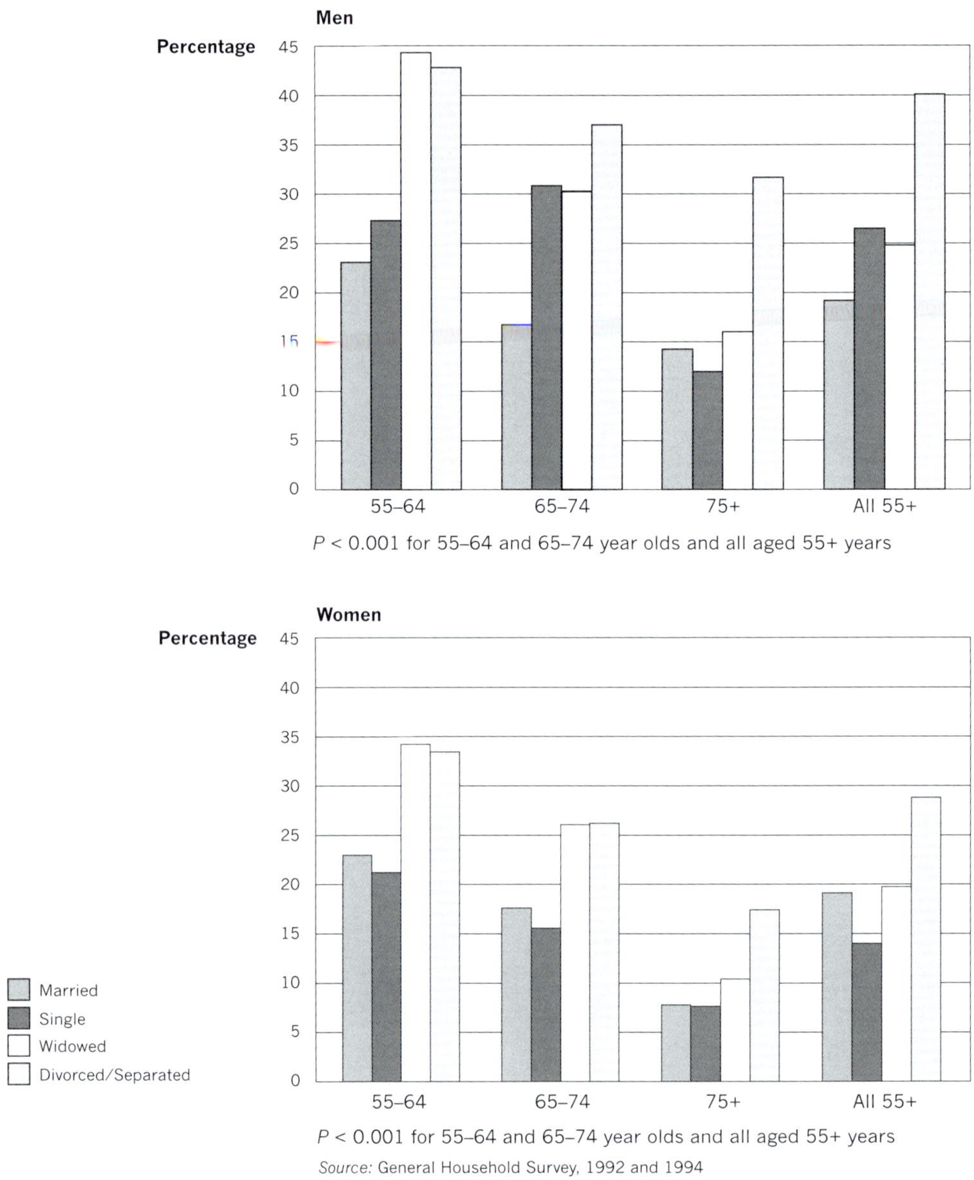

Fig. 3.7. Percentage currently smoking cigarettes by sex, age and marital status

Table 3.1 shows daily cigarette consumption by marital status and examines whether the higher smoking found for divorced/separated men and women also reflects greater cigarette consumption among this group. This was clearly the case for older men, with half of the divorced/separated smokers having 20 or more cigarettes a day, compared with 46% of single men and 38% of married men. Widowed older men were more likely to be moderate smokers than any other group. Older women were less likely to be heavy smokers and more likely to smoke moderately than men regardless of their marital status. Heavy smoking was broadly comparable between married, single and divorced/separated women at around 29%, although the overall level of smoking was much lower for single women than for the divorced/separated and widowed (see Figure 3.7). Similar to older men, older women who are widowed were least likely to smoke heavily, and more likely to be light smokers than single, married or divorced/separated women who smoke.

Table 3.1. Daily cigarette consumption among current smokers by sex and marital status for all aged 55+*

	Married	Single	Widowed	Divorced/separated	All smokers
Men					
Light	24	26	28	21	25
Moderate	38	28	40	29	36
Heavy	38	46	32	50	39
Total (%)	100	100	100	100	100
N =	768	97	167	98	1130
Women					
Light	27	34	36	22	30
Moderate	45	36	42	49	44
Heavy	28	30	22	29	26
Total (%)	100	100	100	100	100
N =	659	56	464	102	1281

Men, P (ns); Women, $P < 0.05$

*Light: 1–9 cigarettes/day; moderate: 10–19 cigarettes/day; heavy: 20+ cigarettes/day

Source: General Household Survey, 1992 and 1994

To summarise, our findings show that the smoking behaviour of older men and women is clearly differentiated according to their socio-economic position, with the most disadvantaged social classes and income groups being more likely to smoke than the higher socio-economic groups. There is some evidence that heavy cigarette consumption is most likely for older men in the bottom income group, whereas the results are more inconsistent for older women who are more likely to be moderate or light smokers. Being divorced is associated with smoking for both sexes, and with heavy smoking for men. A smaller proportion of married men and women are smokers compared with the widowed, and smoking is particularly low among single older women.

Multivariate analysis of cigarette smoking for older men and women

Using logistic regression analysis, it is possible to control for age-related differences in income and living arrangements, which may account for some of the association between these factors and smoking behaviour. It will also determine the extent to which smoking among non-married older people can be attributed to their disadvantaged socioeconomic position. We first present the odds of smoking compared with not smoking, with separate models for older men and women aged 55 and above. The analyses control for age, living arrangements and socioeconomic position. We also include a measure of chronic health status, acknowledging that the presence of 'limiting illness' may influence smoking behaviour.

In order to assess the social determinants of heavy smoking, a further logistic model was computed showing the odds of smoking 20+ cigarettes per day compared with smoking moderately, lightly or not at all. These results are presented in graphical form according to the living arrangements of older men and women after controlling for all of the other variables in the model.

Table 3.2 (Model 1) shows a significant inverse association between smoking and age for both older men and women. The odds of being a smoker for divorced/separated men were twice as high as for married men (the reference category). The odds of smoking were also significantly increased by over 60% for widowed men, whether living alone or with others, relative to the reference category of the maried. Single men living alone had a significantly higher odds ratio of smoking, with the odds for single men living with others being comparable with married men. Widowed women living with others were most likely to smoke, with the odds increased by 88% for this group relative to married women. Similar to older men, being widowed and living alone and being divorced/separated was associated with significantly higher levels of smoking for older women after controlling for age.

For older men and women there was a class gradient in smoking, with the odds of smoking significantly increased for those in manual occupations relative to the professional and managerial group. This was particularly marked for older men, with the odds ratio of smoking increased to 2.27 for the semi- and unskilled class and by 73% for the skilled manual group. Women in manual occupations had their odds of smoking increased by approximately 64% relative to professional and managerial women.

For both sexes, the association between living arrangements and

Table 3.2. Odds ratios for logistic regression of current smoking for men and women aged 55+ years

	Men			**Women**		
	Model 1	**Model 2**	**Model 3**	**Model 1**	**Model 2**	**Model 3**
Age	†††	†††	†††	†††	†††	†††
55–59	1.00	1.00	1.00	1.00	1.00	1.00
60–64	0.81	0.78 *	0.78 *	0.89	0.83	0.83
65–69	0.79 *	0.70 **	0.70 **	0.73 **	0.65 ***	0.65 ***
70–74	0.53 ***	0.44 ***	0.45 ***	0.57 ***	0.48 ***	0.47 ***
75–79	0.57 ***	0.46 ***	0.47 ***	0.39 ***	0.32 ***	0.32 ***
80–84	0.53 ***	0.41 ***	0.42 ***	0.17 ***	0.14 ***	0.13 ***
85+	0.15 ***	0.12 ***	0.12 ***	0.10 ***	0.09 ***	0.08 ***
Living arrangements	†††	†††	†††	†††	†††	†††
Married	1.00	1.00	1.00	1.00	1.00	1.00
Single, live alone	1.48 *	1.13	1.14	1.05	0.93	0.94
Single, live with others	1.03	0.94	0.95	0.55	0.51	0.52
Widowed, live alone	1.65 ***	1.49 **	1.49 **	1.49 ***	1.32 **	1.32 **
Widowed, live with others	1.92 **	2.03 **	2.03 **	1.88 ***	2.02 ***	2.03 ***
Divorced/separated	2.27 ***	1.70 ***	1.71 ***	1.64 ***	1.37 *	1.35 *
Socioeconomic group	†††	†††	†††	†††	ns	ns
Professional and managerial	1.00	1.00	1.00	1.00	1.00	1.00
Routine non-manual	1.30	1.21	1.21	1.13	1.05	1.06
Skilled manual	1.73 ***	1.40 ***	1.40 ***	1.64 ***	1.32	1.32
Semi- and unskilled	2.27 ***	1.69 ***	1.69 ***	1.65 ***	1.25 *	1.24 *
Equivalised household income		††	†		††	†
Top 20%		1.00	1.00		1.00	1.00
60 < 80%		1.09	1.10		1.36 **	1.34 **
40 < 60%		1.29 *	1.28 *		1.48 ***	1.46 **
20 < 40%		1.44 **	1.43 **		1.29 *	1.28
Lowest 20%		1.47 **	1.46 **		1.37 *	1.35 *
Length in current housing tenure		†††	†††		†††	†††
Owner occupier 5+ years		1.00	1.00		1.00	1.00
Owner occupier < 5 years		1.30	1.28		0.79	0.79
Private renter		1.65 **	1.65 **		1.10	1.11
Local auth/housing association 5+ years		1.69 ***	1.70 ***		1.87 ***	1.85 ***
Local auth/housing association < 5 years		2.41 ***	2.42 ***		1.77 ***	1.71 ***
Chronic health status			†			††
No chronic illness			1.00			1.00
Long-standing illness (LI)			0.73 **			0.84
Limiting long-standing illness (LLI)			0.91			1.14
Δ –2LLR	209.4	89.9	8.9	277.9	94.8	9.5
Δ df	14	8	2	14	8	2
N =	4549			5523		

Statistical significance of variable in the model: † $P < 0.05$; †† $P < 0.01$; ††† $P < 0.001$.

Statistical significance of difference from the reference category: * $P < 0.05$; ** $P < 0.01$; *** $P < 0.001$.

Source: General Household Survey 1992 and 1994

smoking behaviour was retained when measures of income and housing were added in Model 2. However, unlike Model 1, the odds of smoking increased for widowed men living with others and decreased for divorced/separated men and widowers living alone relative to the married. Being single and living alone was no longer significantly associated with smoking for older men. A similar trend was seen for older women, with widows living with others over twice as likely to smoke as the married. Divorced/separated women and widows living alone remained significantly more likely to smoke, but the odds decreased for these groups when measures of social class, income and housing were added to the model. This suggests that at least part of the association between smoking and living arrangements results from the disadvantaged socioeconomic position of the divorced, widowed living alone and single older men relative to married couples. Widowed men and women who live with others may have greater access to socioeconomic resources shared by the household, which may explain why the odds of smoking increased for this group when socioeconomic measures were added to the model.

Older men in manual occupations remained most likely to smoke even after controlling for their income and housing, but only older women in the semi- and unskilled class remained significantly more likely to smoke relative to the professional class. For both sexes, equivalised household income was strongly associated with smoking behaviour. For men, those in the lowest income groups were most likely to smoke, with the odds of smoking increased by 47% relative to the reference category. For women, there was a more curvilinear relationship between income and smoking, with the odds ratio of smoking greatest for those in the middle of the income distribution.

After controlling for differences in income, social class and living arrangements, older men and women living in local authority housing were significantly more likely to smoke than those who own their homes. Men living in local authority housing for less than 5 years had the highest odds ratio of smoking, whereas for women the odds ratio was greatest for those who have been in local authority housing for 5 years or more. Living in rented housing was associated with significantly greater smoking among older men but not older women. For both sexes, home ownership is associated with the lowest levels of smoking. These results suggest that smoking is closely associated with material deprivation for older men and older women.

Having a long-standing illness significantly decreased the odds of smoking for older men relative to those without any chronic illness, whereas the odds of smoking for men with an LLI were not signifi-

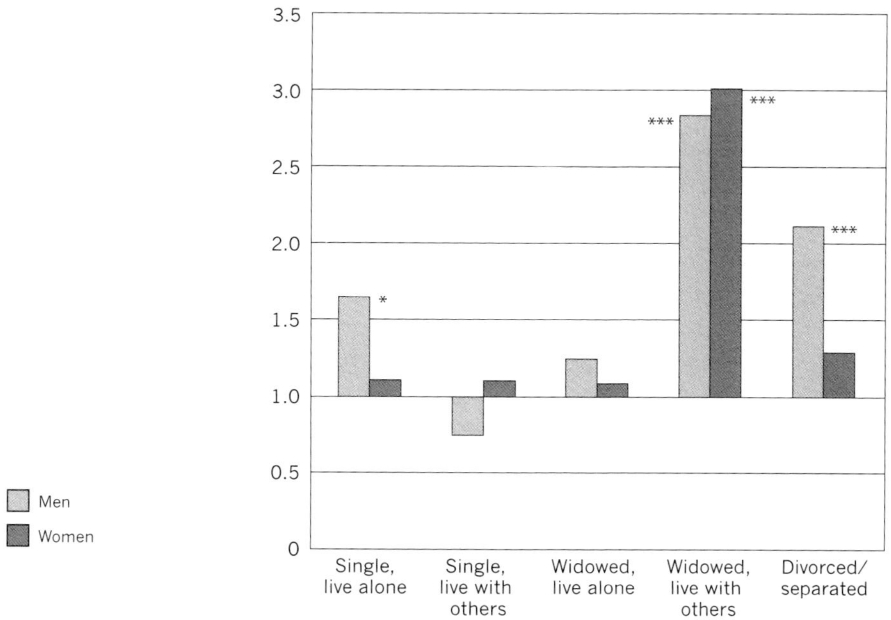

Significance of difference from the reference category: * $P < 0.05$; *** $P < 0.001$
Odds ratios are relative to the married (reference category 1.00)

Source: General Household Survey, 1992 and 1994

Fig. 3.8. Odds ratios of heavy smoking (20+ per day) for older men and women by living arrangements, after controlling for age, socioeconomic position and health status

cantly different from the reference category (Model 3). For women, the measure of chronic health status made a significant overall contribution to the model, but the odds ratios of smoking with an LI and LLI were not significantly different from those with no chronic illness (the reference category).

Turning to the factors which predict heavy smoking, Figure 3.8 shows the odds ratios of heavy smoking (defined as 20 or more cigarettes per day) compared with lighter or non-smokers according to the living arrangements of older men and women after controlling for their socioeconomic position, age and health status. The results confirm that as well as being more likely to smoke (Table 3.2), divorced older men and widowers living with others were more likely to smoke heavily after controlling for the other variables in the model. The odds of heavy smoking were three times as great for widowed men living with others and doubled for divorced men compared with married men. Single men living alone were also significantly more likely to be heavy smokers after accounting for any variation in socioeconomic position between this group and the married. For older women, the odds of heavy smoking were three times higher for widows living with others relative to married women, who were least likely to have a high cigarette consumption. There was some evidence to suggest that divorced/separated older women have an increased likelihood of heavy smoking, but this did not reach statistical significance.

Discussion and conclusions

Our results showed that smoking behaviour was heavily age dependent for men and women, with the oldest age groups being less likely to smoke and less likely to have a high cigarette consumption than younger adults and those in their 50s and 60s. For those aged below 75 years, there was little gender difference in smoking, although men remained more likely to be heavy smokers in each age group. This highlights the importance of controlling for age in any analysis of smoking behaviour and of considering possible cohort differences in lifetime smoking behaviour for men and women.

Consistent with studies based on younger age groups, our results clearly showed the smoking behaviour of older people to be socially patterned. Older men and women in the professional social classes and the highest income groups were least likely to smoke, with smoking strongly associated with socioeconomic disadvantage. These social class inequalities in smoking persist for older age groups despite the fact that many will have left the labour market many years earlier.

Income was strongly associated with smoking after controlling for social class. Smoking among older men consistently increased as their level of equivalised household income decreased, and there was some evidence to suggest that heavy smoking was more likely in the lowest income group. Older women in the highest income group were also least likely to smoke, although the relationship between income and smoking was more inconsistent for women. These findings support other work which shows that smoking is most likely among those social groups who are least able to afford it (Dorsett and Marsh, 1998; Marsh and McKay, 1994). Using cross-sectional survey data, it is impossible to tell whether smoking exacerbates or induces greater financial hardship.

Marital dissolution may bring about adverse changes in income and socioeconomic status, with material resources likely to be divided in the event of divorce or separation (Wyke and Ford, 1992). Our results suggest that at least part of the association between divorce and smoking can be attributed to the less advantaged social position of these groups relative to married couples. However, the higher prevalence of smoking among older people who are widowed and divorced after controlling for socioeconomic factors is a finding which requires further investigation. We do not know whether their smoking behaviour results from the loss of their partner, or whether being divorced or widowed is associated with greater stress or differential social activity. Our results showed that being widowed and living alone was associated with greater smoking for older men and women, and heavy cigarette consumption was found for older men who are divorced or single and living alone. This could suggest that these groups experience greater feelings of isolation or live in poorer socioeconomic circumstances than the married or those living with others, which may prompt their smoking behaviour.

Housing tenure was significantly associated with smoking after controlling for other socioeconomic factors. Local authority housing was associated with greater smoking for both sexes, with older men in rented housing also more likely to smoke than owner occupiers.

Consistent with research on younger age groups (Jarvis, 1994), our results suggest that smoking among older people may increasingly be a marker for material deprivation and poor socioeconomic circumstances. These individuals may experience greater psychological distress than more advantaged social groups, with some evidence that smoking can function to alleviate stress and feelings of isolation among the most socially deprived groups (Graham, 1993; Marsh, 1984). It is therefore important to consider structural factors in understanding why people smoke. For older people who are living on a low income, do not own their home or who are widowed or divorced, smoking may not be so much a matter of personal choice but more a means of coping with adverse social circumstances.

4 The social distribution of high and excessive drinking

Introduction

This chapter examines the drinking behaviour of older men and women aged 55 and above, using data from the GHS and the HSE. We focus on alcohol consumption, in particular the socioeconomic characteristics of those classified as 'high drinkers', and 'excessive drinkers' whose behaviour may be potentially health-damaging.

Previous research has shown that individuals in lower socioeconomic groups are more likely to engage in health-damaging behaviour, such as smoking (Marsh and McKay, 1994; Graham and Hunt, 1994), eating a poor diet (Dowler and Calvert, 1995; Colhoun and Prescott-Clarke, 1996) and lacking physical exercise than those in higher socioeconomic groups. The relationship between socioeconomic position and drinking behaviour is less clear (Uitenbroek, Kevekovska and Festchieva, 1996), and is made more complex by uncertainty about the level of drinking which is detrimental to health – especially for older age groups (Doll, 1997).

Government figures do not consistently show strong social class variation in alcohol consumption, based on drinking over the recommended weekly amount of 21 units for men and 14 units for women (Goddard, 1997; Department of Health, 1996; Bennett *et al.*, 1996). However, levels of alcohol consumption are often presented in these sources as an average for all individuals over the age of 16 years, which may obscure any differences that exist between age groups. This is surprising considering that drinking behaviour is known to be heavily age dependent, with alcohol consumption decreasing markedly with advancing age for men and women (Bennett *et al.*, 1996).

Little is known about the determinants of drinking behaviour within older age groups, for example, how the loss of a partner or living on a low income influences this health behaviour. Adults over the age of 65 are often omitted from studies (for example Uitenbroek, Kevekovska and Festchieva, 1996; Lahelma *et al.*, 1997), or else broad age ranges are used which may conceal the heterogeneity within older age groups and changes in socioeconomic circumstances with advancing age (Goddard, 1997; Department of Health, 1996). By using representative survey data, our study examines levels of alcohol consumption among the over-55s in detail according to their age and socioeconomic position.

By locating the drinking behaviour of older people within a wider socioeconomic context, we can examine the way in which material resources and living circumstances constrain or promote alcohol intake.

Measuring alcohol consumption

The alcohol consumption of individuals is difficult to quantify and measure, with large-scale surveys typically recording a lower level of consumption than would be predicted based on sales of alcoholic beverages (Goddard, 1997). Alcohol consumed at home may be underestimated because the quantity is more imprecisely measured. Levels of drinking are usually classified by units of alcohol consumed, with one unit equivalent to half a pint of beer, a small glass of wine or a single measure of spirits. The 1992 Health of the Nation report (Department of Health, 1992) recommended a weekly 'sensible drinking' limit of 21 units or below for men and up to 14 units for women. More recent government guidelines for 'sensible drinking' are based on a daily limit of between 3 and 4 units per day for men and 2–3 units per day for women (Department of Health, 1995).

Our research classifies alcohol consumption based on the weekly limit, which was applicable at the time the GHS and HSE survey data were collected (further details are given in Appendix B). Men and women drinking over 21 and 14 units respectively are classified as 'high drinkers'. A further threshold is drawn at 51 or more units per week for men and 36 or more units per week for women, representing an indicator of 'excessive drinking' which is more likely to be associated with long-term physical ill-health or psychological damage than 'high' drinking (Royal College of General Practitioners, 1986).

Age-related trends in alcohol consumption

The GHS has consistently shown that alcohol consumption falls with increasing age and is lower for women than for men (Bennett *et al.*, 1996). Results from the 1997 Omnibus survey show that 16–24-year-old men consume an average of 20 units per week, with consumption less than half this level among men aged 65+. For women, these age differences in drinking are even more pronounced, with over one-quarter of older women over 65 years of age drinking no alcohol at all over the last year (Goddard, 1997). However, there is some evidence that within older age groups, high drinking and excessive drinking increased between 1984 and 1994, especially among older men (Bennett *et al.*, 1996).

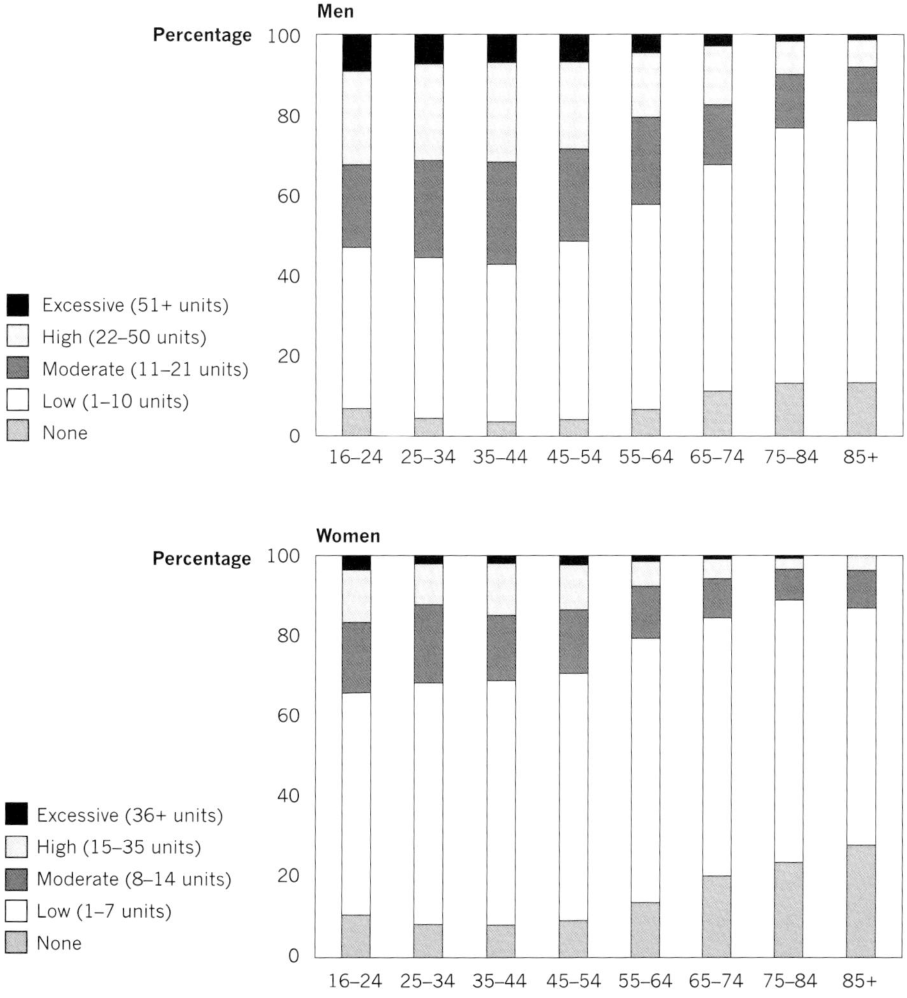

Source: General Household Survey, 1992 and 1994

Fig. 4.1. Levels of weekly alcohol consumption by age group for men and women aged 16+

Figure 4.1 confirms this age-related decrease in alcohol consumption based on two years of GHS data (1992 and 1994). With advancing age, a greater proportion of men and women were non-drinkers, particularly women. Excessive drinking was greatest among the 16–24 age group, and approximately 6% of men drank at this level until their late 50s, when there was a steady decline in excessive alcohol consumption among older age groups. A much smaller percentage of women drank excessively and the proportion of high and excessive drinkers decreased with progressively older age groups.

From cross-sectional data, it is not clear whether people generally drink less as they get older or cohort differences exist in drinking behaviour. Glynn *et al.* (1985) assessed the effects of birth cohort on the alcohol consumption of male volunteers aged between 28 and 82 years who participated in an American longitudinal study of ageing between 1973 and 1984. In both years of the survey, cross-sectional age differences were clearly evident, with older cohorts drinking significantly less in the previous year than younger men. However, over the nine-year time period between surveys, there was no tendency for individual men to decrease their alcohol consumption.

These results suggest that successive generations of older people differ in their drinking behaviour. This is supported by American research showing that people over 75 years of age report different patterns of lifetime drinking behaviour and differ from younger age groups in their attitudes about alcohol and health (Meyers *et al.*, 1981). These generational differences are likely to be gendered, with differing cultural norms concerning appropriate drinking behaviour for men and women of varying ages (Dean, 1989). Goddard (1997) also found strong age differences in drinking-related knowledge, with only 56% of older people aged 65+ having heard about alcohol units, compared with 89% of young people aged 16–24 years.

In addition to cohort differences, the observed decline in drinking with age may also be due in part to a higher mortality rate among long-term heavy drinkers.

Socioeconomic status and alcohol consumption

Results from the 1997 Omnibus survey show that non-drinking is inversely associated with occupational status for all men and women aged 16 and above, with men and women in the lower social classes more likely to be abstainers (Goddard, 1997). No significant class variation in high drinking was found for men, but women in the higher classes were more likely to drink over 14 units a week than those in manual occupations (Goddard, 1997), a finding supported by earlier studies using both individual and household measures of social class (Department of Health, 1996; Goddard, 1991). In 1996, 15% of women in professional and managerial occupations were drinking at a high level compared with 10% in junior non-manual occupations and 8% in the unskilled manual class (Department of Health, 1996). The results show a curvilinear relationship with class for men, with the greatest proportion of high drinkers in the managerial group (29%) and the unskilled manual group (28%) (Department of Health, 1996). 'Harmful' or excessive drinking has been found to be comparable across all social classes for men and women, although none of these studies control for age (Goddard, 1997; Department of Health, 1996).

The failure to find consistent socioeconomic variation in drinking behaviour amongst the general adult population has led some to conclude that alcohol consumption is not socially patterned in the UK (Royal College of General Practitioners, 1986). However, using income as a measure of socioeconomic position for all adults aged 16+, there is evidence that men living in high-income households (over £500 per week) are more likely to exceed the sensible drinking limit than those in households with low incomes below £100 per week (Bennett *et al.*, 1996). For women, the association between household income and high drinking is more marked, ranging from 19% of women in households with high income to 9% in low-income households. These results suggest that, unlike other health-damaging behaviour, the propensity to drink alcohol is greater among the more affluent social groups who have the economic resources to purchase alcohol and maintain a higher level of alcohol consumption (Uitenbroek, Kevekovska and Festchieva, 1996), but these studies have not controlled for age.

Goddard (1991) examined whether life stage influenced alcohol consumption by analysing information on age, marital status and age of youngest child from the 1987 and 1989 OPCS surveys on drinking behaviour. Although these studies included older people, the sampling procedure used favoured younger respondents below 45 years of age and the analyses did not control for age amongst those who were divorced and widowed. The results showed that single men and women under 30 years of age were most likely to be high drinkers (over 21 units per week), with alcohol consumption also high among divorced men (34%) and divorced women (14%). Amongst the widowed, 16% of men were high drinkers compared with only 3% of women. Figures from the Department of Health (1996) confirm that divorced men are more likely to exceed sensible drinking levels than married men. For both sexes, widowhood was associated with the lowest levels of alcohol consumption (Department of Health, 1996).

There is some evidence that divorced men of all ages are more likely to drink over 50 units per week, with the levels of harmful drinking observed for divorced men being comparable with young single men (Goddard, 1991).

Greater psychological distress has been reported among single and widowed men and divorced women compared with their married counterparts, which could suggest that marriage has an integrative effect which may positively influence health behaviour. Umberson (1992) found evidence that women are likely to monitor their spouses' health and health-related behaviour. Based on American survey data from adults over 24 years of age, married men were more likely to report this 'social control' on their behaviour than the unmarried, whereas negative health behaviour (including higher alcohol consumption) was associated with divorce. Married women did not report significantly more attempts by others to monitor their health behaviour than non-married women, suggesting that marriage has more of a health protective effect for men than for women. However, in a study of drinking patterns among older Americans, Barnes (1979) found no evidence that widowhood was associated with increased levels of problem drinking for older men or women.

These findings suggest that alcohol consumption is influenced by marital status and socioeconomic position, although the interpretation of many of these results is problematic, because the analyses do not control for underlying age differences. As with smoking, the perceived benefits of drinking alcohol often include relaxation (Hall *et al.*, 1992), stress relief and social activity (Royal College of General Practitioners, 1986), but unlike smoking, evidence suggests that high alcohol consumption is more prevalent amongst higher socioeconomic groups. Excessive drinking may reflect a dependency on alcohol (so-called 'problem drinking') which may differ in its social distribution from high drinking. Figures suggest that excessive drinking is more prevalent among divorced men and women, but there is a need to examine the relationship between marital status and both high and excessive drinking among different age groups.

Aims

The use of large-scale data in our study will allow us firstly to distinguish levels of alcohol consumption within older age groups and secondly to examine the socioeconomic characteristics of older people who exceed the recommended 'sensible drinking' levels of 21 units per week for men and 14 units per week for women. In particular we focus on the living circumstances of these 'high drinkers' to investigate whether the loss of a partner through death or divorce influences alcohol intake for older men and women. For widowed and never married older people, we distinguish between those living alone and those living with others, (the small numbers of divorced/separated older men and women meant that it was not possible to distinguish their living arrangements in this way). We can therefore try and assess whether isolation or loneliness may be a factor in understanding their drinking behaviour.

Within this 'high drinking' group of older people, we then separate out those with an 'excessive' alcohol intake (51+ units for men and 36+ units for women) from older people who are high but not excessive drinkers. Our analysis mainly uses GHS data to compare the social distribution of excessive and high (but not excessive) drinking for men and women aged 55+ according to their age, living circumstances, social class and income. Using the HSE data, we have constructed an index of personal deprivation (see Appendix A) to reflect differences in the material living conditions of older people which may also influence their drinking behaviour.

Multivariate logistic regression analysis is used to examine the relative contribution of these social factors to the drinking behaviour of older people, and to highlight any variation according to gender and marital status.

Differences in alcohol consumption within older age groups

Figure 4.2 shows current levels of alcohol consumption among five-year age groups of older people aged 55+ using data from the GHS for 1992 and 1994 combined. Women were more likely to be non-drinkers than men, and for both sexes the proportion of non-drinkers increased with age. This was especially marked for women, with 30% of those aged 85+ not drinking any alcohol in the previous week compared with 14% of women in their late 50s. The majority of older men and women consumed a low or moderate amount of alcohol regardless of their age, with 54% of men and 62% of women aged 55 and above drinking low levels of alcohol. High drinking decreased markedly with age for men and women. Nearly three times more men and four times more women in their late 50s drank this amount compared with the oldest age group aged 85 and above.

Excessive drinking was very low and was also inversely related to age for both sexes. The proportion of men drinking at this level fell from 5% in the 55–59 age group to 2% of 70–74-year-olds and only 1% of men aged 85+ years. For women, less than 1% of those over the age of 70 years exceeded 35 units of alcohol per week.

A similar trend in alcohol consumption was found using data from the HSE (Table 4.1), although reported levels of high and excessive drinking were generally somewhat higher than in the GHS.

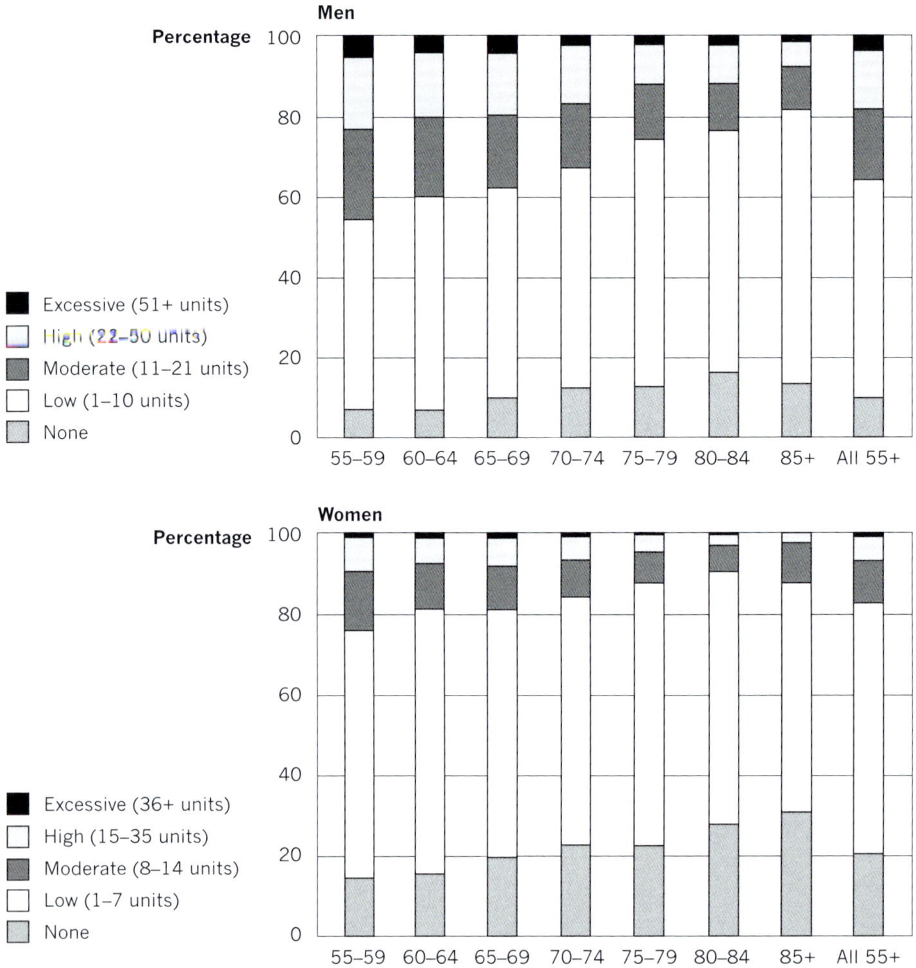

Source: General Household Survey, 1992 and 1994

Fig. 4.2. Levels of weekly alcohol consumption by age group for men and women aged 55+

Table 4.1. Comparison of the percentage of high and excessive drinkers in the GHS and HSE data for older men and women

	Men						
	55–59	**60–64**	**65–69**	**70–74**	**75–79**	**80+**	**All 55+**
High (22–50 units)							
GHS	17.9	16.0	15.5	14.7	10.2	8.7	14.7
HSE	22.4	18.9	17.8	14.1	13.2	8.4	17.0
Excessive (51+ units)							
GHS	5.1	3.9	4.0	2.0	1.7	1.7	3.4
HSE	6.8	4.4	5.2	2.9	2.3	0.2	4.2
	Women						
	55–59	**60–64**	**65–69**	**70–74**	**75–79**	**80+**	**All 55+**
High (15–35 units)							
GHS	8.8	6.3	7.3	6.3	4.5	2.7	6.2
HSE	12.1	8.6	8.9	6.8	7.2	4.7	8.2
Excessive (36+ units)							
GHS	1.0	1.4	1.0	0.7	0.4	0.3	0.9
HSE	0.9	1.1	1.3	0.8	0.7	0.6	0.9

Source: General Household Survey, 1992 and 1994; Health Survey for England, 1993 and 1994

Socioeconomic determinants of 'high drinking' within older age groups

We now examine social variation in drinking within 10-year age groups of older men and women. Figure 4.3 shows the percentage drinking above the recommended weekly amount of 21 units for men and 14 units for women by socioeconomic group.

For men in their late 50s and early 60s, broadly comparable levels of drinking were observed for those in professional and managerial occupations and the semi- and unskilled class. In the 65–74-year age group, nearly one-quarter of men in the highest social class had a high alcohol intake, which decreased markedly for men in routine non-manual occupations (12%) and rose to around 16% among men in the semi- and unskilled social class. From age 75 upwards, there was clearer evidence of class variation in alcohol consumption, with professional and managerial men much more likely to drink at a high level than those in junior non-manual and manual occupations. The proportion

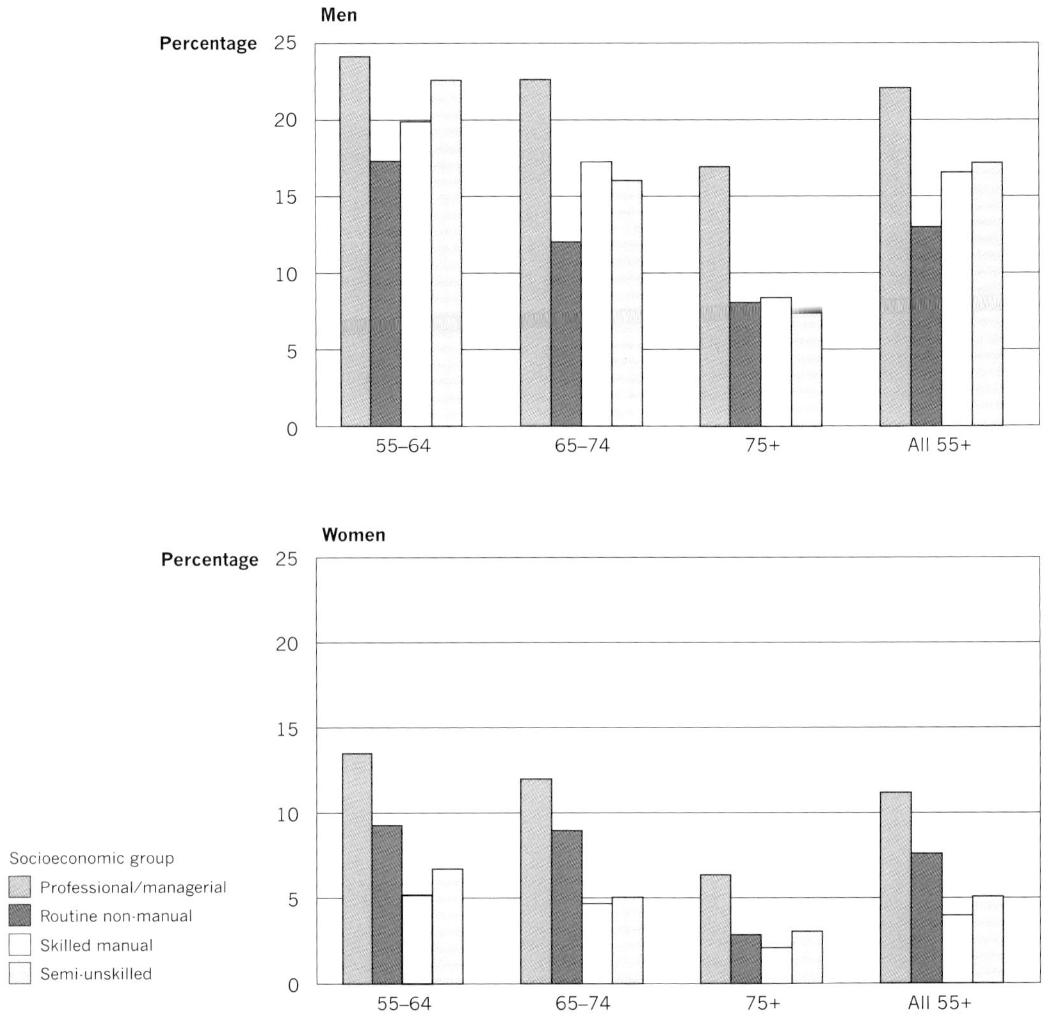

Source: General Household Survey, 1992 and 1994

Fig. 4.3. Percentage drinking over recommended weekly amount (22+ units for men and 15+ units for women) by age and socioeconomic group

of high drinkers decreased from 17% of professionals to approximately 7% of older men in manual social classes.

Unlike for men, professional and managerial women aged 55–64 years were much more likely to exceed recommended drinking levels, with alcohol consumption more than halved among semi- and unskilled women in comparison. These strong class differences persisted among older age groups of women, although the number of women with a high alcohol intake decreased markedly for all social classes.

Similar results were found for older women based on their

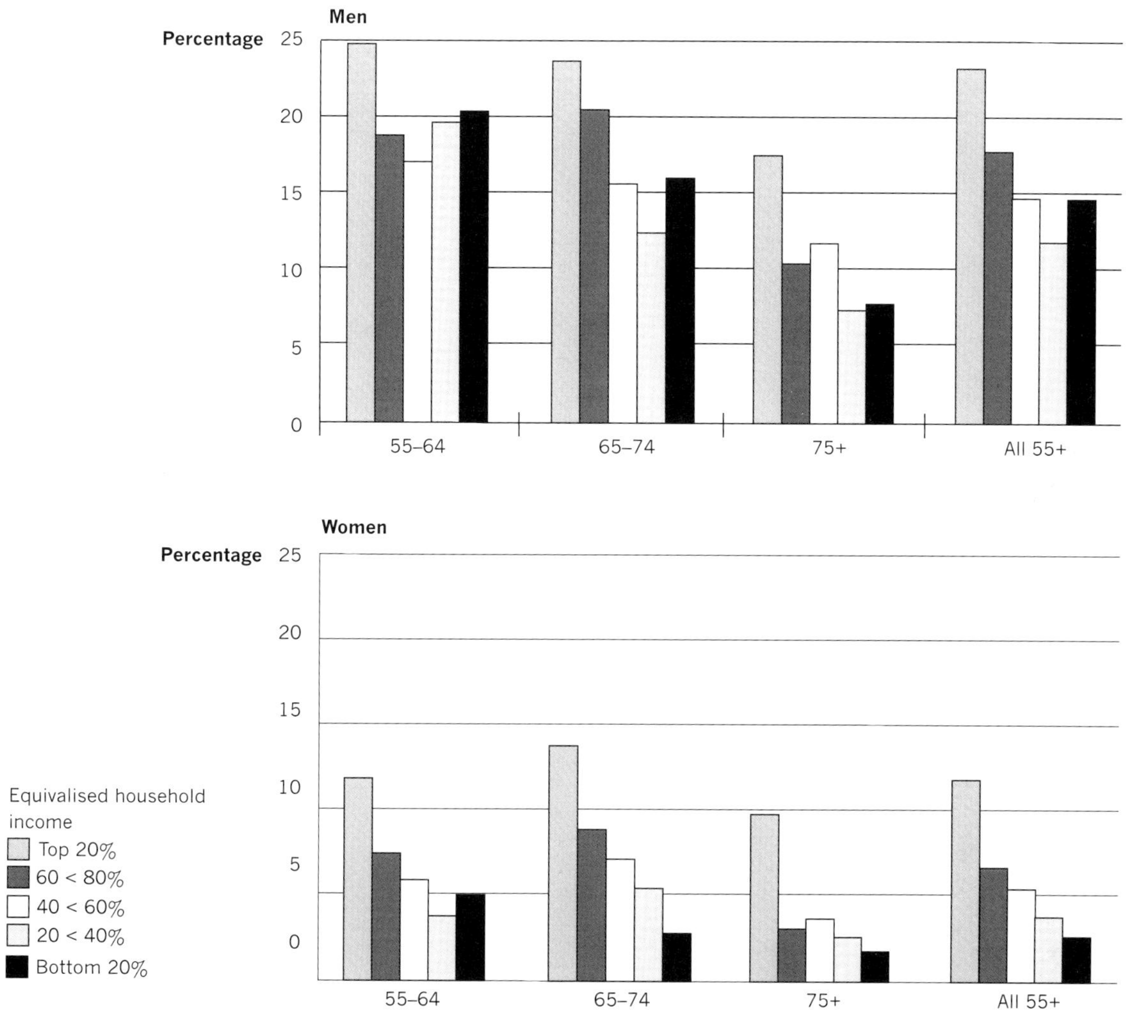

Source: General Household Survey, 1992 and 1994

Fig. 4.4. Percentage drinking over the recommended weekly amount (22+ units for men and 15+ units for women) by age and equivalised household income

equivalised household income (Figure 4.4), with those in the top 20% of the income distribution having the highest levels of drinking. For women aged 65–74 years, the proportion of high drinkers fell from 14% in the top quintile to 3% in the lowest income group. Older men in the highest income group were also most likely to have a high alcohol intake, with the income gradients in drinking becoming more pronounced in older age groups. This suggests that financial resources are important in facilitating high levels of drinking.

When drinking behaviour was examined by marital status the results

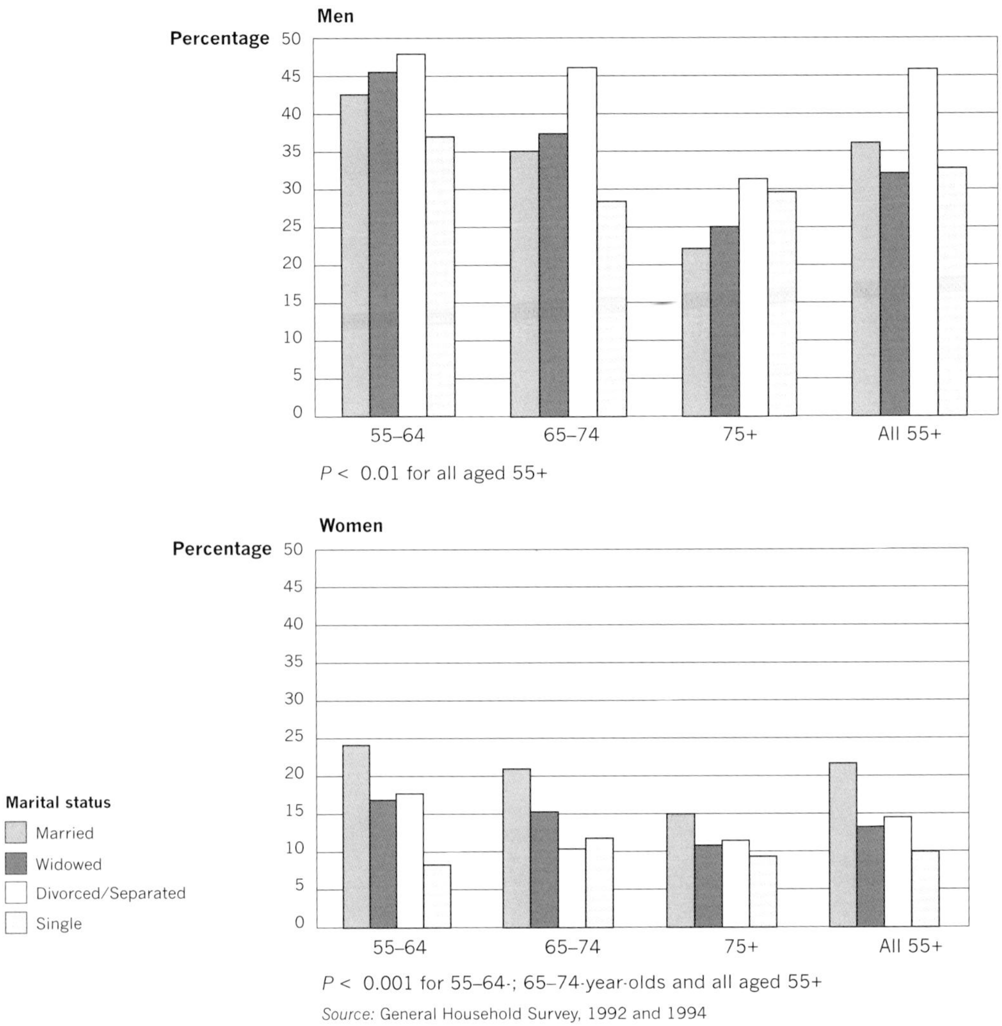

Fig. 4.5. Percentage drinking over the recommended weekly amount (22+ units for men and 15+ units for women) by age and marital status

showed that, for men, drinking was greatest among the divorced/separated, with approximately 45% aged 55+ having a high alcohol intake (Figure 4.5). Drinking was substantially lower for single men below 75 years of age, and more widowed men in these age groups drank at a high level than married men. For those aged 75+, approximately 30% of divorced and single men were high drinkers, which fell to 25% of widowers and was lowest among the married. Therefore there were different patterns of high drinking according to marital status and this varied according to age among men over 55 years.

In contrast, divorced women in each age group had lower levels of drinking than married women. For women aged 55–64 and 75+, the widowed and divorced had broadly comparable levels of drinking, and high drinking was least likely for older single women. For the 65–74-year age group, a greater proportion of widows were high drinkers than divorced or single women, but their level of drinking remained well below that observed for married women.

To summarise our findings for men and women aged over 55 years, the higher social classes and income groups were more likely to be high drinkers than lower socioeconomic groups. For older women, clear socioeconomic differences in drinking were evident from age 55 upwards, whereas for men the gradients in high alcohol consumption were more pronounced among the oldest age groups. The relationship between marital status and alcohol intake clearly differed for older men and women. Within each age group, being divorced was associated with the highest levels of drinking for men, whereas married women were most likely to have a high alcohol intake. In the following section, we apply a higher drinking threshold of 51+ units and 36+ units for men and women respectively to compare the social characteristics of older people with an excessive alcohol intake which is likely to be damaging to health, compared to those with a high (but not excessive) level of alcohol consumption.

Socioeconomic determinants of 'high' and 'excessive' drinking

These results assess social variation in alcohol consumption when an 'excessive drinking' threshold is applied to those older people consuming over the recommended weekly amount of alcohol. Figure 4.6 distinguishes between older people drinking at an 'excessive' level of over 50 units for men and over 35 units for women and those who exceed the recommended threshold (over 21 units for men and above 14 units for women) but do not have an excessive alcohol intake. For both sexes, alcohol consumption was greatest among the professional and managerial class, with 18% of men and 10% of women drinking at a high but not excessive level. Older men in routine non-manual jobs were least likely to be high drinkers (11%), with the proportion drinking at this level slightly higher at 13% for those in manual occupations. For women there was a more consistent decrease in alcohol consumption with decreasing social class. Alcohol consumption for older women in manual groups was less than half that observed among professional and managerial women.

For excessive drinking, there was no difference between older men in the highest and lowest social classes, with approximately 4% of professional and unskilled manual men drinking at this level, falling to half

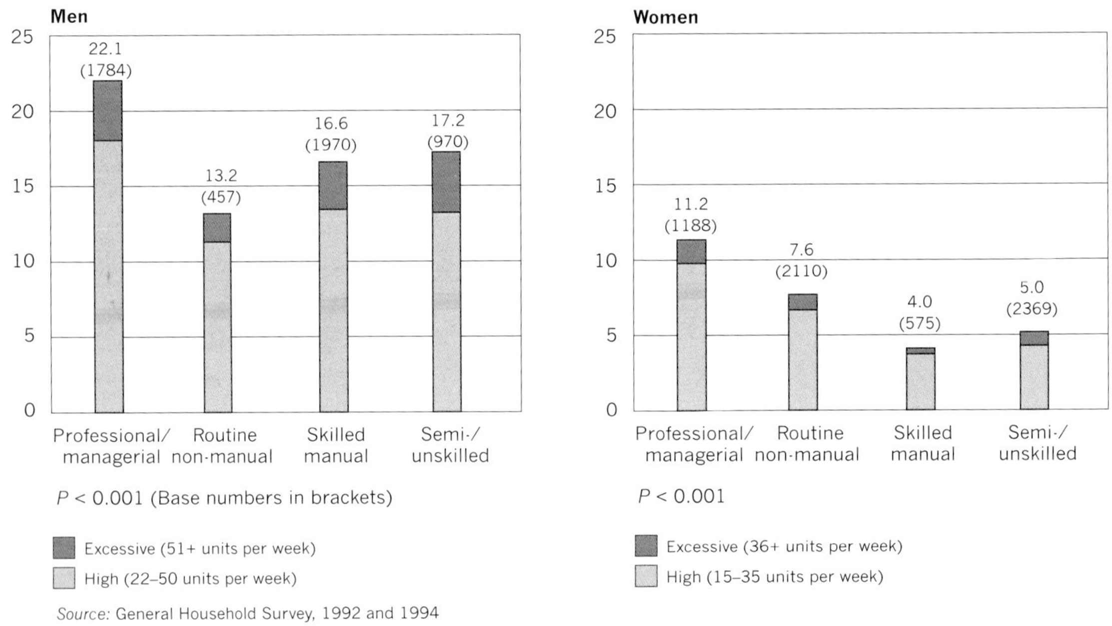

Fig. 4.6. Percentage with alcohol consumption above recommended level by socioeconomic group for men and women aged 55+

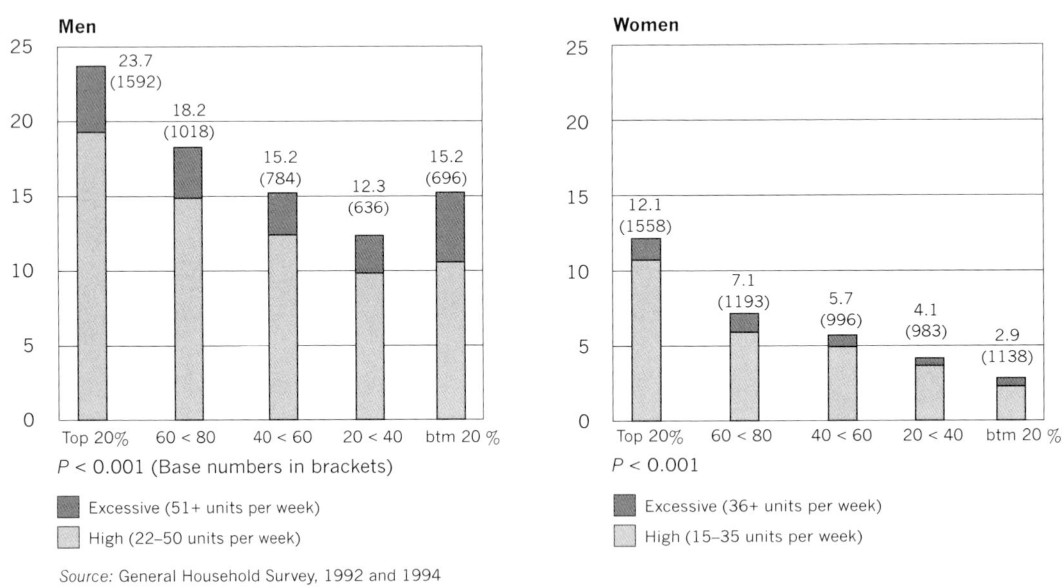

Fig. 4.7. Percentage with alcohol consumption above recommended level by equivalised household income for men and women aged 55+

this level among men in the junior non-manual group. For women, only a very small proportion drank over 35 units per week, but there was some evidence that this was greater within the professional and managerial class (1.4%).

Figure 4.7 examines levels of high and excessive alcohol consumption by equivalised household income, divided into quintiles. Men in the top 20% of the income distribution were more likely to have a high alcohol intake than any other income group. There was also a greater level of high drinking among the lowest income group relative to the second lowest quintile, and the proportion of excessive drinkers in this group was comparable to the top income group at 4.5%. For older women, there was a clear inverse association between high drinking and level of income, with 10% of high drinkers in the top income quintile compared with 5% in the middle of the distribution and only 2% in the lowest income group. The proportion of excessive drinkers also decreased with decreasing income among women.

These income results are stronger than those found using social class, and support previous research which suggests that income is likely to determine the ability to purchase alcohol on a regular basis. There is some evidence that the relationship between excessive alcohol consumption and socioeconomic position varies according to gender. For older men, the association between excessive drinking and socioeconomic position was a curvilinear one, with the highest and lowest income groups comparable in their levels of very high drinking. A more consistent decrease in excessive drinking was found for older women as their household income decreased.

When we used the HSE data to examine the relationship between material deprivation and alcohol intake (based on our constructed Index of Personal Deprivation – see Appendix A), a strong gradient in high drinking was found for older women, but the results were again more curvilinear for older men (Figure 4.8). Women living in the least deprived circumstances (score 0) were four times more likely to have a high level of drinking than those who were most deprived. For men, roughly equivalent levels of high drinking were found for those with a PDI score of 0 and 3. Those in the most deprived group (PDI score of 4) were most likely to be excessive drinkers. In the most disadvantaged groups, 10% of older men drank 51 or more units per week, which was more than double the proportion of excessive drinkers seen in any other group. The PDI index differs from the other measures of socioeconomic position used in our analysis in that it provides a measure of material and financial resources, such as car ownership, home ownership and receipt of Income Support. It may therefore be a more precise

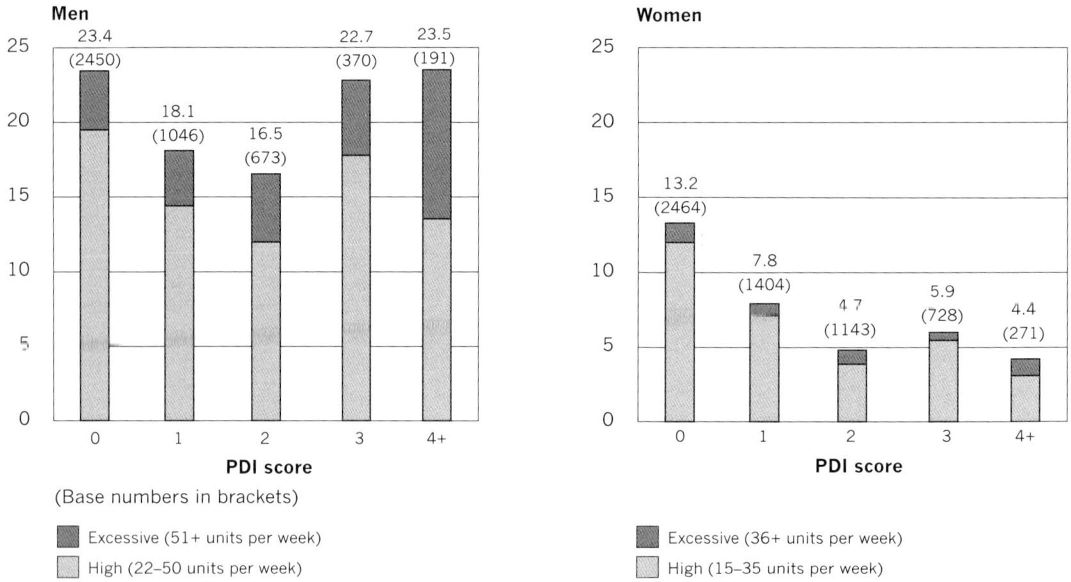

Source: Health Survey for England, 1993 and 1994

Fig. 4.8. Percentage with alcohol consumption above recommended level by personal deprivation index (PDI) score for men and women aged 55+

indicator of the relationship between current living circumstances and drinking behaviour than measures of social class or income.

The living arrangements of older people were significantly associated with their drinking behaviour, but in a different way for men and women (Figure 4.9). Results from the GHS showed that 27% of older divorced/separated men drank over the recommended limit, compared with approximately 17% for single and widowed men. The divorced group contained the largest proportion of excessive drinkers at 9%, followed by single men at 6.3%, and excessive drinking was lowest among older widowed and married men. There was no evidence that living alone is associated with higher alcohol intake among single and widowed men, since comparable levels of high and excessive drinking were found in these groups for those who live alone or with others.

For women, the married had the highest levels of alcohol consumption at 9%, followed by the divorced/separated (8%), and these two groups contained the greatest proportion of excessive drinkers. For women there was more variation in alcohol consumption according to whether they lived alone or with other people. Widows who live alone showed slightly increased levels of high drinking compared with widows who live with other people, whereas for single older women, living

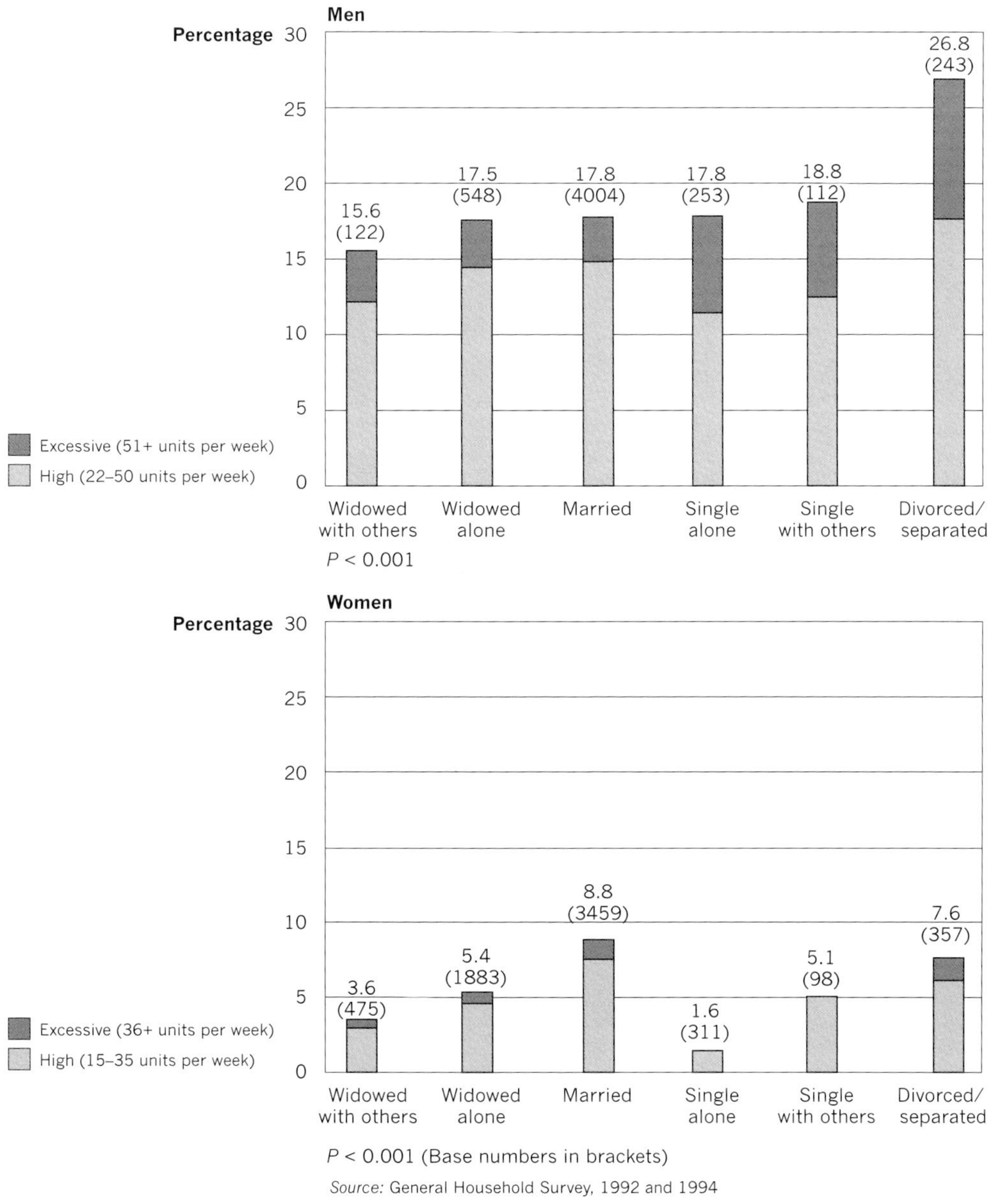

Fig. 4.9. Percentage with alcohol consumption above recommended level by living arrangements for men and women aged 55+

alone was associated with the lowest levels of alcohol consumption. No single older women were found to drink at an excessive level.

Our results show that clear social differences exist in high and excessive drinking behaviour, and this varies for older men and older women. For men, excessive or 'problem drinking' was greater in the highest and lowest social classes and income groups and was most strongly associated with deprived living conditions. For women there was a decrease in excessive drinking with worsening socioeconomic position. High drinking was more prevalent among higher socioeconomic groups for both sexes, particularly for older women. Divorce was associated with high and excessive levels of drinking for older men and women, but there was little difference between divorced and married women in this regard. Single older men were more likely to drink excessively.

Our results suggest that lack of economic resources may be important in determining levels of excessive alcohol consumption among men. Long-term excessive drinking or dependency on alcohol may impair individuals' ability to work, earn a living and maintain relationships. Downward mobility, for example, through job loss or marital breakdown, among persistently heavy drinkers may account for the increasing proportion of excessive drinkers seen in the lowest socioeconomic groups and among the divorced. However, cross-sectional data cannot identify the direction of causality between excessive drinking and deprivation. It may also be that the stresses of living in highly deprived social and economic circumstances lead to excessive drinking, but this only appears to be the case for older men and not for older women.

Multivariate analysis of high and excessive drinking for men and women

Drinking behaviour among older age groups is socially patterned. It is important to examine in more detail the relative contribution made by social class, income and living arrangements to the likelihood of drinking above the recommended limit. The lower alcohol consumption observed among single older women, for example, may be a consequence of greater financial constraints experienced by this group relative to married women. We therefore proceed with a logistic regression analysis which presents the odds for all older people drinking over the recommended weekly amount of 21 units for men and 14 units for women compared with alcohol consumption below this limit. Models are presented separately for older men and women to highlight any gender differences in drinking behaviour after controlling for age, living arrangements and socioeconomic position. We also include measures of current smoking behaviour and chronic health status, acknowledging that current drinking behaviour may be influenced by the presence of 'limiting' ill health and by the tendency to engage in other health-damaging behaviour. However, we cannot determine the direction of causation between smoking, health and drinking using cross-sectional data.

In order to assess whether the social determinants of 'excessive' drinking (defined as 51+ units for men and 36+ units for women) differ from those for 'high' drinking, a logistic model is presented in the following section for older men showing the odds of drinking more than 50 units per week. Owing to the small numbers involved, it was not possible to undertake this logistic regression analysis for older women.

Drinking above the recommended limit for men and women aged 55+

Table 4.2 (Model 1) shows a significant inverse association between age and drinking above the recommended limit for older men and women. Divorced/separated men had a 50% higher odds of this level of drinking compared to the married. Widowed men who live alone were also significantly more likely to be high drinkers, with widowed men living with others and single men living alone being comparable with the reference category of married men. For women, the married were most likely to drink above the recommended level, with the odds ratios of this level of drinking substantially reduced for single older women living alone, and halved for widowed women living with others.

For both sexes, the association between drinking above the recommended level and living arrangements was strengthened when measures of socioeconomic position were added in Model 2. For men, the odds of high drinking increased to 61% for the divorced/separated and to nearly 50% for widowers living alone relative to married men after controlling for any variation associated with their income, social class and housing tenure. Single women living alone had their odds of high drinking significantly reduced by 87% relative to the married, with widows living with others also remaining less likely than married women to have a high alcohol intake. These results do not suggest that underlying socioeconomic differences can account for the variation in alcohol consumption associated with the living circumstances of older people.

Controlling for socioeconomic position improved the overall fit of the model by 96.3 for women compared with 54.6 for men. For both sexes, those in the professional and managerial class were most likely to drink above the recommended level. In comparison, those in the semi- and unskilled class had their odds of high drinking reduced by 25% for men and 38% for women. Men in routine non-manual occupations were least likely to have a high level of alcohol consumption, with the odds halved for this group in comparison to the professional and managerial class. For older women, there was a consistent decrease in the odds of high drinking as income level decreased, with those in the lowest income group having their odds of high alcohol intake significantly

Table 4.2. Odds ratios for logistic regression of drinking above the recommended limit‡ for men and women aged 55+ years

	Men			Women		
	Model 1	**Model 2**	**Model 3**	**Model 1**	**Model 2**	**Model 3**
Age	†††	†††	†††	†††	††	ns
55–59	1.00	1.00	1.00	1.00	1.00	1.00
60–64	0.85	0.90	0.90	0.77	0.85	0.86
65–69	0.81	0.91	0.90	0.94	1.18	1.22
70–74	0.67 ***	0.78 *	0.75 *	0.73	0.99	1.05
75–79	0.42 ***	0.49 ***	0.49 ***	0.53 **	0.75	0.85
80–84	0.42 ***	0.49 ***	0.49 ***	0.26 ***	0.38 **	0.50 *
85+	0.17 ***	0.20 ***	0.20 ***	0.31 **	0.45 *	0.65
Living arrangements	†	††	††	††	††	†††
Married	1.00	1.00	1.00	1.00	1.00	1.00
Single, live alone	0.98	1.06	1.14	0.14 ***	0.13 ***	0.12 ***
Single, live with others	1.28	1.37	1.43	0.63	0.59	0.68
Widowed, live alone	1.40 *	1.49 **	1.51 **	0.77	0.95	0.88
Widowed, live with others	1.05	1.03	0.97	0.50 *	0.47 **	0.42 **
Divorced/separated	1.50 **	1.61 **	1.57 **	0.82	1.09	1.01
Socioeconomic group		†††	†††		††	††
Professional and managerial		1.00	1.00		1.00	1.00
Routine non-manual		0.49 ***	0.46 ***		0.71 *	0.69 **
Skilled manual		0.75 **	0.72 ***		0.56 *	0.52 ***
Semi- and unskilled		0.75 *	0.71 **		0.62 **	0.59 ***
Equivalised household income		††	†††		†††	†††
Top 20%		1.00	1.00		1.00	1.00
60 < 80		0.83	0.82		0.65 **	0.62 **
40 < 60		0.69 **	0.67 **		0.60 **	0.56 ***
20 < 40		0.57 ***	0.55 ***		0.48 ***	0.45 ***
Bottom 20%		0.68 **	0.64 **		0.35 ***	0.34 ***
Housing tenure		ns	ns		††	†††
Owner occupier		1.00	1.00		1.00	1.00
Rented		1.01	0.94		0.94	0.89
Local authority housing association		1.09	0.98		0.57 ***	0.51 ***
Smoking status			†††			†††
Never smoked cigarettes			1.00			1.00
Ex-cigarette smoker			2.26 ***			2.29 ***
Currently smoke cigarettes			2.52 ***			3.03 ***
Chronic illness			ns			ns
No chronic illness			1.00			1.00
Long-standing illness (LI)			1.04			1.12
Limiting long-standing illness (LLI)			0.94			0.89
Δ -2LLR	79.9	54.6	77.4	86.4	96.3	73.7
Δ df	11	9	4	11	9	4
N =	4539			5521		

‡ defined as over 21 units/week for men and over 14 units/week for women

Statistical significance of variable in the model: † $P < 0.05$; †† $P < 0.01$; ††† $P < 0.001$

Statistical significance of difference from reference category: * $P < 0.05$; ** $P < 0.01$; *** $P < 0.001$

Source: General Household Survey, 1992 and 1994

reduced to nearly one-third relative to the highest income group. For older men, the odds ratios of drinking above the recommended level were decreased as income fell, but were slightly higher for the bottom income group relative to the second lowest income quintile.

Housing tenure was not significantly associated with high alcohol consumption for older men, but older women living in local authority housing were significantly less likely to be high drinkers than those who owned their own home. This suggests that the socioeconomic position and the living environment of older women is important in determining their level of alcohol consumption.

Although having an LLI lowered the odds of drinking above the recommended level for older men and women compared to those with no chronic illness, these results did not reach statistical significance after controlling for the other factors in the model (Model 3). There was no evidence that the lower alcohol consumption of widows living with others, for example, can be attributed to the greater ill health of this group.

Smoking behaviour was strongly associated with drinking for both sexes after controlling for age, health status and socioeconomic position. Older men who smoked had 2.5 times higher odds of drinking above the recommended level than those who had never smoked, whilst for older women the odds were three times greater. For both men and women, ex-smokers were over twice as likely to drink at a high level than the reference category of never smoked.

The differences in alcohol consumption by living arrangements shown in Model 1 were not due to differences in socioeconomic position, health status or smoking, since Model 3 shows that clear differences remained in the alcohol consumption of older men and women according to their living arrangements when these other variables were included in the model. Figure 4.10 presents a graph of these odds ratios using the married as the reference category (1.00). The figure shows that, for older men, living alone was associated with increased odds of high drinking relative to married men, although this was only statistically significant for lone widowers and for men who were divorced/separated. The high proportion drinking above the recommended level among older divorced/separated men and older widowers who live alone cannot be explained by their poorer socioeconomic and financial circumstances. Non-married older women were less likely to drink above the recommended level than married women, and this was statistically significant for single women living alone and widowed women living with others.

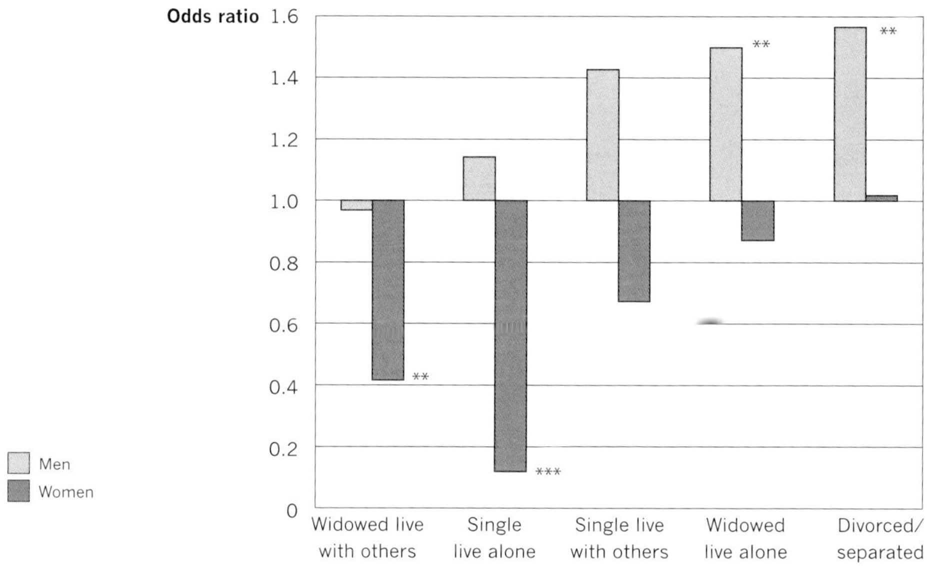

Significance of difference from the reference category: ** $P < 0.01$ *** $P < 0.001$
Odds relative to the married (reference category = 1.00)
Source: General Household Survey, 1992 and 1994

Fig. 4.10. Odds ratios of drinking above the recommended level (defined as 22+ units for men and 15+ units for women) for older men and women by living arrangements, after controlling for age, socioeconomic position and health status

Excessive drinking for men aged 55+

When the odds of drinking excessively (51+ units per week) were examined for men, there was a significant age-related decrease in excessive alcohol consumption (Table 4.3; Model 1). Unlike drinking above the recommended level, the likelihood of excessive drinking was substantially higher for single as well as for divorced/separated older men. Single men living alone had over twice the odds of drinking excessively compared with married men, whilst single men living with others had an odds ratio 2.5 times greater. This could suggest that single (never married) men have different lifetime drinking behaviour to their married or previously married counterparts. Widowers living alone, who were significantly more likely to exceed recommended drinking levels, also had a higher odds ratio of excessive drinking. The odds of excessive alcohol intake were over three times greater for divorced/separated older men than for married men after controlling for age. Married older men were therefore the group least likely to be excessive drinkers.

Men in the professional and managerial class were most likely to drink 51+ units per week, with the odds of excessive drinking significantly reduced for those in routine non-manual occupations in comparison. There was some evidence of a curvilinear relationship between income and excessive drinking, with men in the lowest income group having slightly increased odds of drinking at this level compared with the highest income quintile, but these results were not statistically significant. As with drinking above the recommended level, housing tenure was not significantly associated with excessive drinking for older men, although the odds were increased for those living in rented housing relative to the reference category of owner occupiers. Adding socioeconomic measures to the model slightly lowered the odds of excessive drinking found for the divorced/separated and single, but these men remained substantially more likely to drink at this level than the married.

The strong relationship between smoking and drinking above the recommended level (Table 4.2) was also evident for excessive drinking among older men (Table 4.3). The odds of excessive drinking were over three times higher for current smokers and increased twofold for ex-smokers compared with the reference category of those who had never smoked.

As with drinking above the recommended weekly limit, chronic illness was not significantly associated with drinking at an excessive level. However, the odds of having an excessive alcohol intake did increase for those with a reported LI or LLI relative to those with no chronic ill health. Using cross-sectional data it is impossible to interpret whether persistent excessive drinking causes chronic ill health among older men, or whether the presence of chronic illness exacerbates increased dependency on alcohol.

Discussion and conclusions

Our results showed clear age-related differences in alcohol consumption in later life, both between younger and older age groups and within older age groups for men and women, which highlights the importance of accounting for age in any study of drinking behaviour.

The social determinants of alcohol consumption among older age groups differed according to whether drinking was defined as high (more than 21 units for men and over 14 units for women) or excessive (51+ units for men and 36+ for women). For both sexes, high drinking was most prevalent among the higher social classes and the wealthiest income groups. There was a more linear decrease in high alcohol consumption for older women as their socioeconomic position decreased, whereas for older men there was a slight upturn in high drinking among the poorest income group and the unskilled social class. This

Table 4.3. Odds ratios for logistic regression of excessive drinking‡ for men aged 55+

	Model 1	Model 2	Model 3
Age	†††	†	†
55–59	1.00	1.00	1.00
60–64	0.79	0.82	0.81
65–69	0.82	0.90	0.89
70–74	0.45 **	0.49 *	0.50 *
75–79	0.35 **	0.38 *	0.39 *
80–84	0.35 *	0.37 *	0.39 *
85+	0.12 *	0.12 *	0.14
Living arrangements	†††	†††	††
Married	1.00	1.00	1.00
Single, live alone	2.03 *	1.88 *	1.97 *
Single, live with others	2.58 *	2.53 *	2.70 *
Widowed, live alone	1.63	1.61	1.58
Widowed, live with others	1.60	1.60	1.41
Divorced/separated	3.13 ***	2.89 ***	2.66 ***
Socioeconomic group		ns	ns
Professional and managerial		1.00	1.00
Routine non-manual		0.43 *	0.40 *
Skilled manual		0.77	0.73
Semi- and unskilled		0.88	0.81
Equivalised household income		ns	ns
Top 20%		1.00	1.00
60 < 80		0.88	0.82
40 < 60		0.71	0.64
20 < 40		0.67	0.59
Bottom 20%		1.14	1.01
Housing tenure		ns	ns
Owner occupier		1.00	1.00
Rented		1.45	1.34
Local authority housing association		1.18	0.97
Smoking status			†††
Never smoked cigarettes			1.00
Ex-cigarette smoker			2.28 ***
Currently smoke cigarettes			3.31 ***
Chronic illness			ns
No chronic illness			1.00
Longstanding illness (LI)			1.28
Limiting longstanding illness (LLI)			1.42
Δ –2LLR	50.2	12.4	26.5
Δ df	11	9	4
N =	4539		

‡ defined as 51+ units/week for men

Statistical significance of variable in the model: † $P < 0.05$; †† $P < 0.01$; ††† $P < 0.001$.

Statistical significance of difference from reference category: * $P < 0.05$; ** $P < 0.01$; *** $P < 0.001$.

Source: General Household Survey, 1992 and 1994

curvilinear relationship between socioeconomic position and alcohol consumption above the recommended level for men was seen more clearly for excessive drinking, which was comparable between the highest and lowest social classes and income groups. This higher level of excessive alcohol consumption among the poorest group of older men could suggest that their disadvantaged living circumstances prompt drinking which acts as a 'coping mechanism' in much the same way as smoking has been shown to function (Marsh and McKay, 1994; Graham and Hunt, 1994).

The results suggest that financial resources are important in maintaining a high alcohol intake, but that in the most disadvantaged social circumstances excessive alcohol consumption may be used as a coping mechanism. However, our measure of average weekly alcohol consumption gave no indication of patterns of drinking, such as the number of alcoholic beverages drunk on any one occasion. The average alcohol consumption of the higher socioeconomic groups may be greater because their drinking is more evenly distributed over the one-week reference period than for lower socioeconomic groups. Little is known about social variation in patterns of drinking, especially among older age groups, and the implications of 'binge drinking' or drunkenness for the health and health promotion of this age group.

Current living arrangements interacted with gender to influence drinking behaviour. Older married men were least likely to drink at a high or excessive level, whereas for older women, marriage was associated with the highest levels of alcohol consumption. The finding that married men were least likely to drink above the recommended level could suggest that men's health behaviour is monitored to some extent by their spouse. For single, widowed and divorced/separated men, the absence of a partner to facilitate positive health behaviour may account for their increased alcohol consumption. There is also evidence to suggest that men living alone experience greater psychological distress than their married counterparts (Cramer, 1993) and that stress associated with marital dissolution may itself prompt a higher alcohol intake (Umberson, 1992). Non-married older women have lower levels of alcohol consumption than the married. These women may be more likely to monitor their own health status, hence marriage may not be such an important control on behaviour as it is for men. Indeed, there is some evidence to suggest that drinking habits of women are negatively influenced by their spouse, with women who drink heavily likely to be married to heavy drinkers (Jacob and Seilhamer, 1982).

The finding that widowed women had lower levels of drinking than married women suggests that patterns of high alcohol consumption cease after the death of a spouse. Functional disability may prompt older men and women who are widowed to live with others. The alcohol intake of this group may therefore be limited by their health status, particularly for older women. However, both of these explanations must remain speculative, as it is not possible to examine any changes in drinking behaviour associated with widowhood or deterioration in health using cross-sectional data. Only longitudinal data can determine more clearly how changes in marital status and living arrangements and health status may influence the alcohol consumption of this age group.

There was a strong association between smoking and drinking behaviour, with older men and women who were smokers or ex-smokers significantly more likely to drink above the recommended level after controlling for their age, socioeconomic position and health status. This 'clustering' of health-damaging behaviour is an implicit assumption of many studies which construct indices of 'risky lifestyles' (Pill, Peters and Robling, 1993), but the strength of the association between smoking and alcohol consumption has rarely been demonstrated specifically for older age groups. In a study based on middle-class adults aged 18–60 years, Burrows and Nettleton (1995) found evidence that professional male smokers drank significantly more alcohol per week than smokers in any other socioeconomic group.

More research is needed to examine the social characteristics of older people who exceed recommended drinking guidelines or who sustain an excessive level of alcohol consumption. Our study suggests that this is more likely among the higher socioeconomic groups who may have greater financial resources to maintain this lifestyle than the lower socioeconomic groups, but that excessive drinking in particular occurs among non-married men who are living in socially disadvantaged circumstances.

5 Physical activity: recreational, home-based and walking

Introduction

Physical exercise has been shown to promote health in a number of ways (Fentem, Bassey and Turnbull, 1988; Fentem, 1992) and the benefits apply also to older people (Haskell, 1997; Pescatello and DiPietro, 1993; Edwards and Larson, 1992). It can help maintain bone density and mobility, diminishing the risk of osteoporosis, falls and fractures (Department of Health, 1994; King and Tinetti, 1995; Gibson, 1990), maintain musculoskeletal integrity (Isdale, 1993), reduce obesity and blood pressure, diminish the risk of cardiovascular disease and stroke (Morris, 1994; Blumenthal *et al.*, 1989; World Health Organization, 1995) and improve mental functioning (Baylor and Spirdoso, 1988; Emery and Gatz, 1990; Rogers, Meiper and Mortel, 1990). Physical activity may help prevent viral infections and certain cancers (Fentem, 1992; Council of Europe, 1995).

Exercise interacts with diet, as a recent Antarctic expedition demonstrated (Stroud, 1998); strenuous exercise by the participants increased their fat metabolism so that a diet with four times the recommended consumption of saturated fats did not raise cholesterol levels. Moreover, older people often eat insufficient food to ensure adequate levels of micro-nutrients. Exercise allows food intake to be increased without the danger of weight gain which would result if the lifestyle were sedentary.

Physical activity also has more general therapeutic effects, being associated with psychological wellbeing, enabling enjoyment of the full range of leisure activities and improving the capacity to respond to the challenges of everyday life (Council of Europe, 1995).

It is a paradox that while public health has benefited from improved nutrition and hygiene, mechanisation of production and increased car ownership has dramatically reduced the amount of muscle power required in work and in travelling. Increasingly sedentary lives incur a health risk unless compensated for by regular exercise. While an increasing proportion of the population of Europe do engage in sport and physical recreation, those who do not are becoming less and less fit, jeopardising their health and bringing 'a dramatic slide in average fitness levels' (Council of Europe, 1995, p. 2). Because 'physical inactivity is probably the most prevalent modifiable health risk factor' (p. 13) 'promotion of exercise is at the very core of positive public health strategy' (p. 11).

For older people, physical fitness is crucial to maintaining functional independence; managing the activities of daily living without assistance depends on having an adequate power–weight ratio and a sufficient degree of joint flexibility. Women's lower average power–weight ratio, combined for some with arthritis, makes them more prone to restricted mobility than men, with an associated loss of functional ability and independence (Arber and Ginn, 1991). Older women are more vulnerable to bone fractures than men and a relatively inactive lifestyle is a contributory factor. For example, hip fracture is twice as common among inactive as active individuals (Council of Europe, 1995, p. 19), owing to both poorer postural control and weaker bones among the inactive. As older people approach the limit of their strength in performing the activities of daily living, ordinary tasks may precipitate failures, strains and falls. The spare muscular and aerobic capacity developed through exercise can lessen the risk of such trauma.

A substantial proportion of people over the age of 50 are judged to take insufficient exercise, in that their physical activity is not of adequate frequency, duration and intensity to produce a health benefit (Skelton *et al.*, 1998). These authors found a difference between men and women in muscular strength within each five-year age group; for example, men had a 20-year advantage over women in the ability to mount steps or rise from a low chair without using their arms (Skelton *et al.*, 1998). This is likely to reflect both sex-linked genetic effects and gender differences in lifetime physical exercise habits.

The reasons for older people's low level of exercise were explored in a recent qualitative study (Finch, 1997). Although older people recognised the value of physical exercise to health, barriers to exercise included a perceived lack of suitable facilities for older people; lack of transport or money; physical restrictions due to illness; lack of time; a fatalistic attitude to health, especially among men; and a strong perception that physical activity could endanger health 'at our age'. For example, an increased heart rate or breathlessness was perceived as risky.

Confidence in the physical capability to engage in exercise, termed 'exercise self-efficacy' (Clark, 1996, p. 157) has been shown to be an important factor in older people's willingness to engage in physical activity. For adults of all ages, exercise self-efficacy depends on absence of disabling conditions, previous positive experiences of physical activities, prevalence of appropriate role models and verbal encouragement by others (Clark, 1996). Since older people's previous experiences of physical recreational activities may be related to their class background, their type and level of physical activity are likely to vary with social class, as well as with their current health status. Possession of adequate material resources may also influence older people's opportunities for exercise, as participation in recreational activities often incurs costs.

In this chapter, two years of the HSE, 1993 and 1994, were combined to examine physical activity among men and women aged 55 and over. We chart the variation in physical activity according to gender, age group, marital status, health, class, educational level and material resources. We assess whether lack of resources, low educational level or low social class is a more important correlate of inactivity, the extent to which poor health restricts physical activity compared with age, and how gender and marital status influence the type or amount of activity.

The HSE questions on activity and exercise are similar to those in the Allied Dunbar Fitness Survey (Activity and Health Research, 1992; Skelton *et al.*, 1998), including recreational activities, domestic work, gardening/DIY and walking. We analyse five kinds of physical recreational activities – cycling, swimming, dancing, aerobics and exercises; activities in which less than 1 per cent of people aged over 55 participated – weight training, running/jogging, football/rugby, badminton/tennis and squash and other – are not reported here. The HSE records frequency of participation in each kind of activity in the previous four weeks and also provides an indication of the effort expended, or intensity of activity; for example, the pace of walking and the type of housework is recorded (see Appendix C). In the analysis we use two HSE-derived variables, one measuring the level (or intensity) of total physical activity, including both recreational and functional activities, the other summarising both intensity and frequency. We use the HSE measures of moderate and vigorous activity (implying energy use of at least 5 kcals/min), while bearing in mind that the same activity level may reflect different amounts of effort and have different significance for health, depending on age and gender.

We first analyse older people's participation in various types of physical activity according to age, gender and marital status, before turning to the effects of resources.

Effects of age, gender and marital status

Physical recreation

The proportions of men and women aged 55 and over who had participated in cycling, exercises (sit-ups or press-ups), swimming, dancing and aerobics during the past four weeks are shown in Figure 5.1.

The rates of participation in each of these five activities were low; however, 32% of men and 26% of women participated in at least one

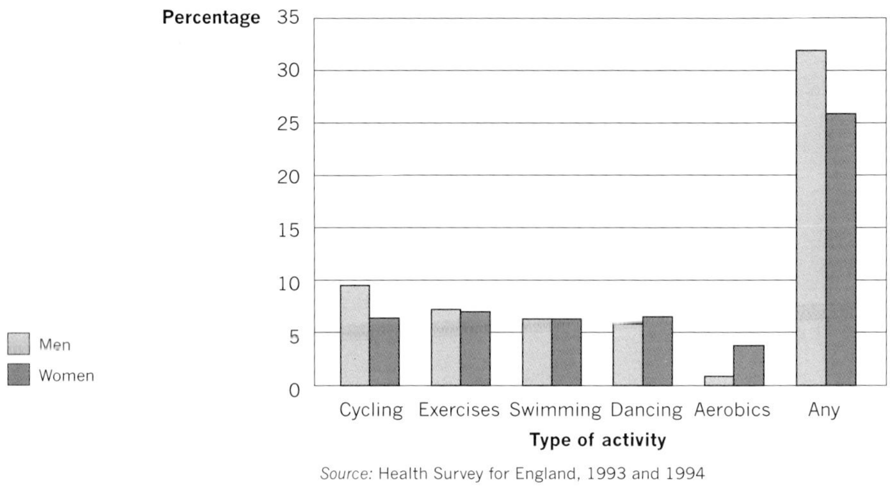

Fig. 5.1. Percentage participating in each recreational activity in the past four weeks: men and women aged 55+

physical recreational activity ('any'). 'Any' activity includes, in addition to the five activities, less popular activities, such as weight training, running, tennis, squash, badminton and other sporting activities, but not walking. Gender differences within type of activity were only evident for cycling, reported by 9.6% of men but 6.4% of women, and aerobics, reported by only 0.8% of men but 3.7% of women. The gender difference in aerobics attendance highlights the question of perceptions as to the gender-appropriateness of activities, which may inhibit one gender from participating.

Figure 5.2(a) shows the proportions of men and women in five-year age groups who participated in any physical recreational activity and Figure 5.2 (b–f) shows participation in each of the five main types of activity by age group. The decline with age in the proportion participating in any activity is clear for women, falling linearly from 40% in the youngest age group, 55–59, to 8% among those aged over 80 (see Figure 5.2(a). For men, there is little sign of decline in their participation rate until age 70. A gender difference is evident after age 65, when women's recreational activity was less than men's in each age group.

Turning to the separate activities – for cycling, swimming and aerobics, women's participation rate declined linearly with age group, while for dancing the age-related decline applied only after age 65 and for exercises (sit-ups and press-ups) only after age 70. Men's participation rate was less clearly related to age. For example, men's highest rate of cycling was among those aged 60–64 and for dancing and exercises was in the age group 65–69. The tendency for men's participation rate to rise with age before falling may be related to

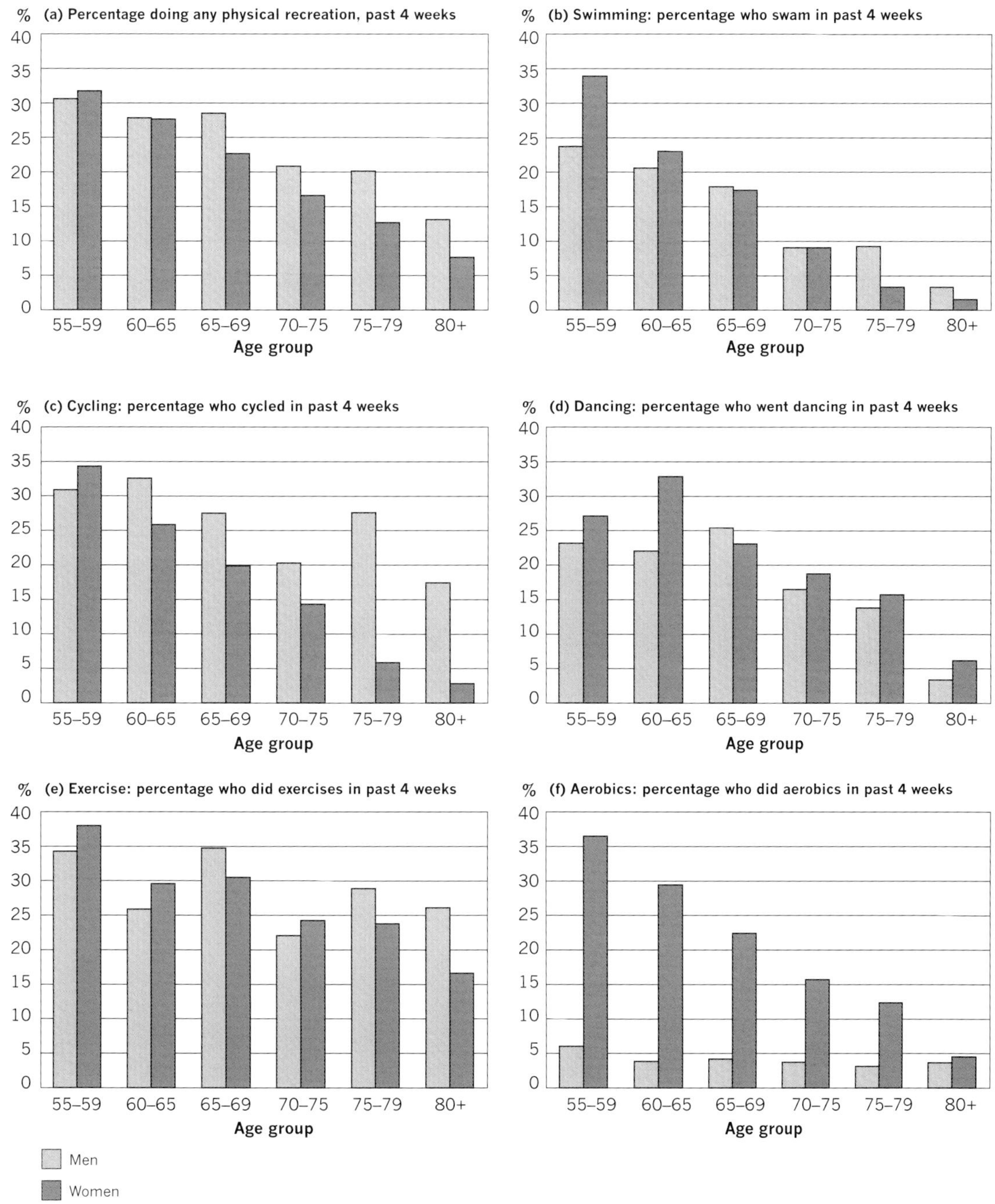

Source: Health Survey for England, 1993 and 1994

Fig. 5.2. Percentage participating in various recreational activities in the past four weeks by gender and age group

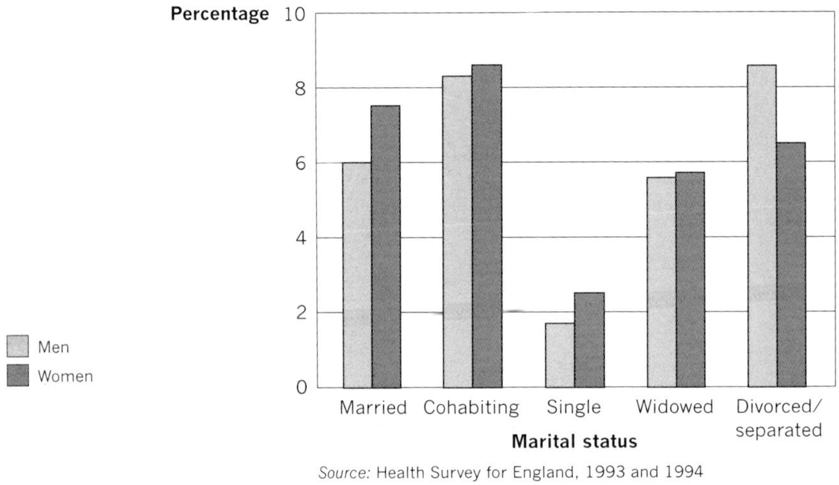

Fig. 5.3. Percentage who went dancing in past four weeks by marital status: men and women aged 55+

cessation of paid employment, releasing time and energy for other activities. Women's increased likelihood of dancing between age 60 and 64 may reflect their own retirement or the increased availability of male partners as husbands and friends retire.

Participation in dancing varied according to marital status (see Figure 5.3). Single people were much less likely than others to go dancing; less than 2% of single people, compared with 6% of married men and nearly 8% of married women, went dancing in the previous four weeks. However, divorced men were the group most likely to have been dancing. These differences may reflect differences earlier in the life course, with single people less likely to have acquired the ability to dance.

Walking

Although often experienced as an enjoyable and sociable leisure activity, walking differs from the above activities in being also a part of normal functioning in daily life. Requiring no special equipment, time-keeping, transport, money or arrangements with others, walking provides an easy and convenient way to improve health, by strengthening muscles and, if the pace is brisk enough, improving aerobic capacity. The HSE provides information on ability to walk at all, whether the individual has walked at least one mile in the past four weeks, frequency of such walks and usual pace of walking.

Figure 5.4 shows the proportion of men and women who had walked at least one mile in the past four weeks, subdivided into those whose usual pace was slow or steady and those whose pace was brisk or fast, by five-year age groups. The proportion who had walked at least a

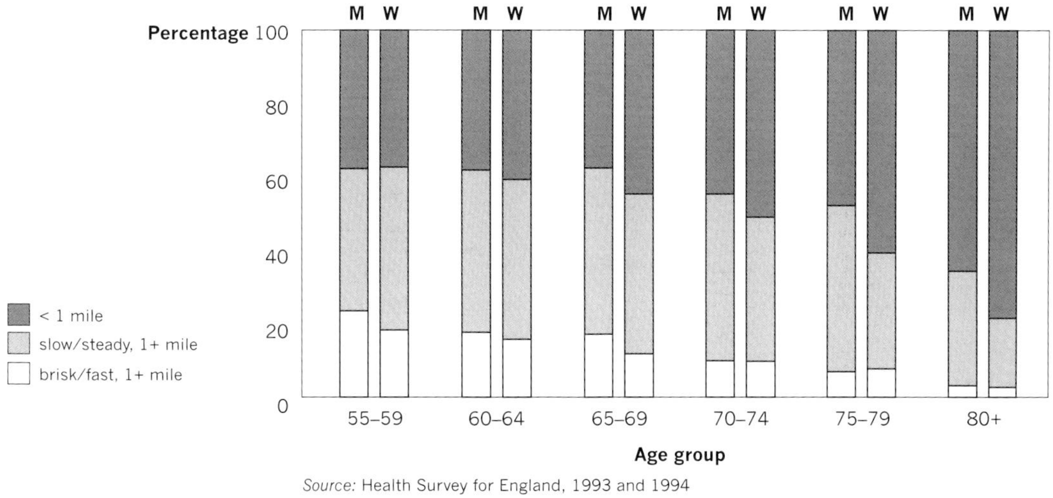

Fig. 5.4. Percentage who walked 1+ mile in past four weeks and usual pace, by gender and age group

mile at a brisk or fast pace declined with age and was less than 10% for all those aged 70 or over. The proportion walking at least a mile, at any pace, declined from 62% of men and women aged 55–59 to 35% of men and 22% of women aged over 80. A noticeable gender divergence emerged after age 65, with women's walking decreasing more steeply than men's. For men, the proportion walking at least a mile showed no decline until age 70.

Figure 5.5 shows the frequency of walking in the past four weeks. There was no decline in men's frequency of walking until age 70. The proportion of men who took walks of at least a mile, at least ten times, rose slightly from 27% at age 55–59 to 30% from 60–69, before declining to just under 26% at age 70–74. Women's frequency of walking declined more linearly with age.

Domestic work

Work done in the home varies in the physical effort required, ranging from dusting to floor-scrubbing. Accordingly, the HSE distinguishes between light and heavy housework (see Appendix C). Although light housework, including such tasks as food preparation, cooking, laundry and so on is generally insufficient to improve aerobic capacity, it is nevertheless likely to be more beneficial to health than inactivity, in that it maintains blood circulation and joint mobility. Heavy housework, which includes Spring cleaning, moving furniture, cleaning windows, carrying heavy shopping for at least five minutes and scrubbing floors, requires more physical effort, thus maintaining muscular strength and, with long enough duration, aerobic capacity as well.

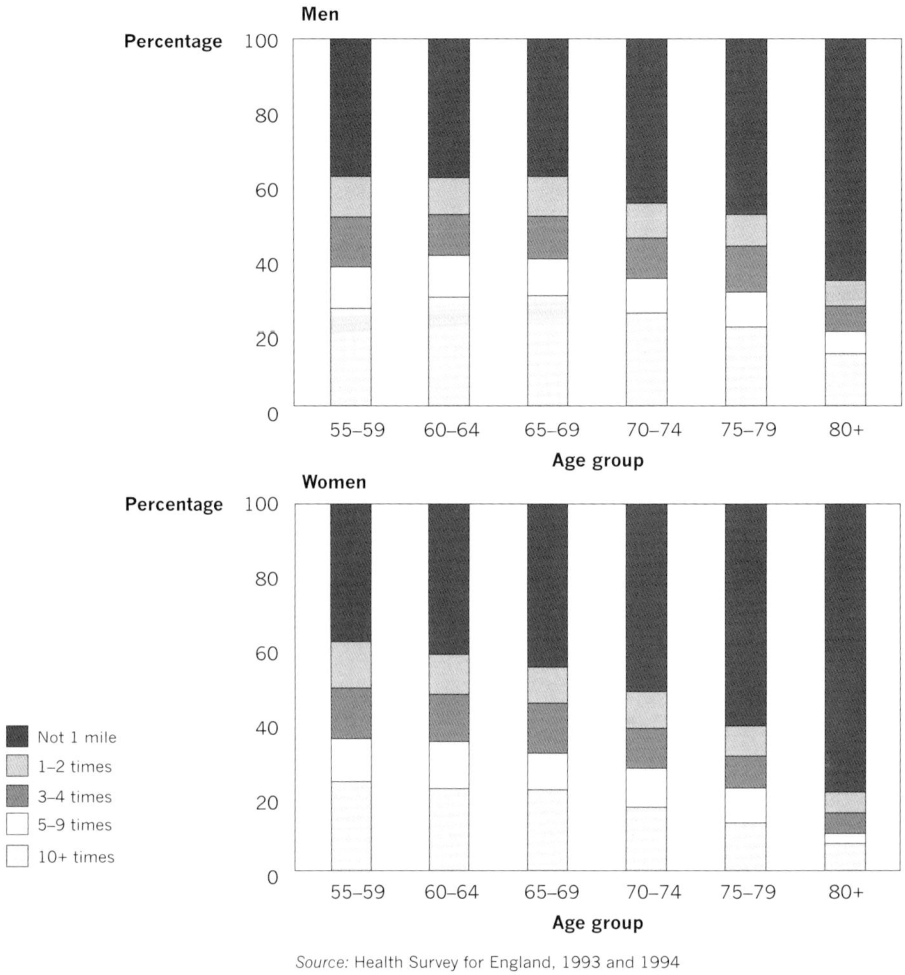

Fig. 5.5. Walking 1+ mile, frequency in past four weeks by gender and age group

Figure 5.6 shows the frequency and intensity of men's and women's domestic work in the past four weeks by age group. Not surprisingly, given the gendered norms as to the division of labour and men's later average age at retirement, women did more housework than men. For example, among women aged 55–59, nearly all (99%) did some housework, a quarter did only light housework and three-quarters did heavy housework; 16% of these women had done heavy housework more than ten times in the past four weeks. Among men in this age group, about 80% did some housework but less than half did heavy housework and only 5% had done heavy housework more than ten times in the previous four weeks.

However, gender convergence with age was evident; whereas women's performance of domestic work declined linearly with age, in

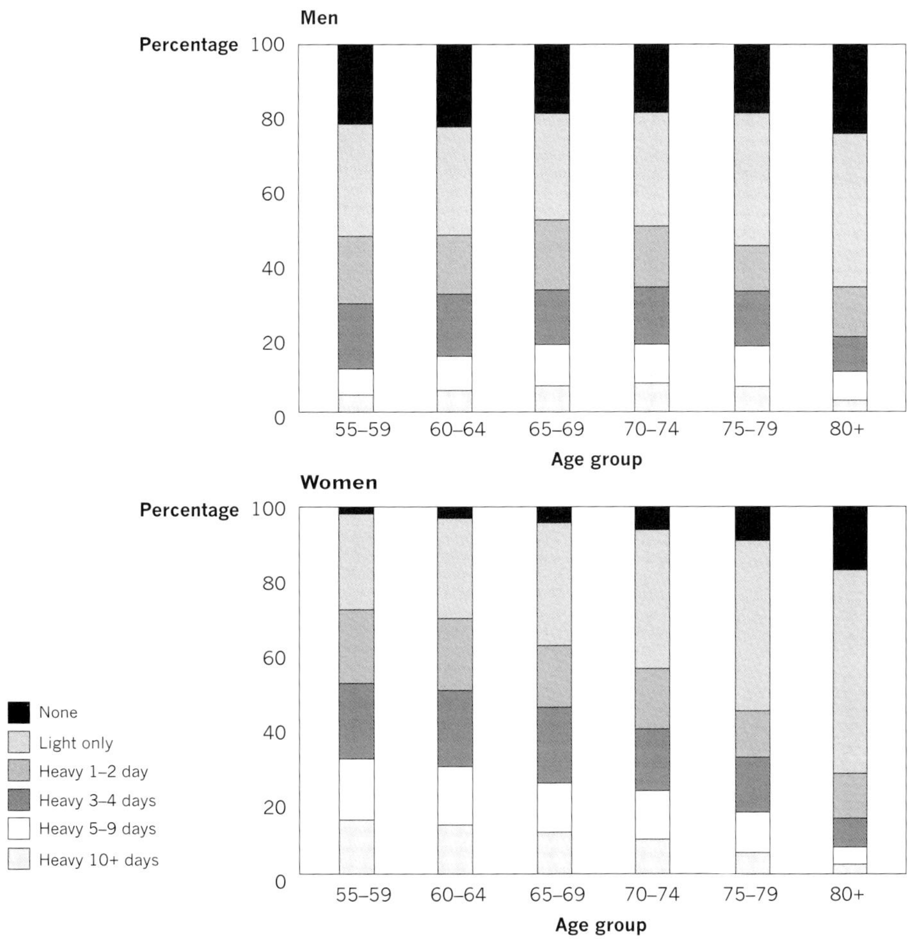

Source: Health Survey for England, 1993 and 1994

Fig. 5.6. Domestic work: frequency in past four weeks and intensity by gender and age group

each category of intensity and frequency, men's did not. Indeed, the proportion of men doing any housework increased slightly after age 65 to 81%, only declining after age 80. The proportion of men doing heavy domestic work was highest from age 65–74, at just over 50%. By age 75, women's dominance in the performance of heavy domestic work had disappeared and by age 80 there was very little gender difference in the proportion doing any housework. The gender convergence in housework is likely to be partly due to men's increased presence in the home after retirement, making a more equal division of domestic labour possible. It may also reflect widening gender differences with age in prevalence of disability (Arber and Ginn, 1991; Arber and Cooper, 1998).

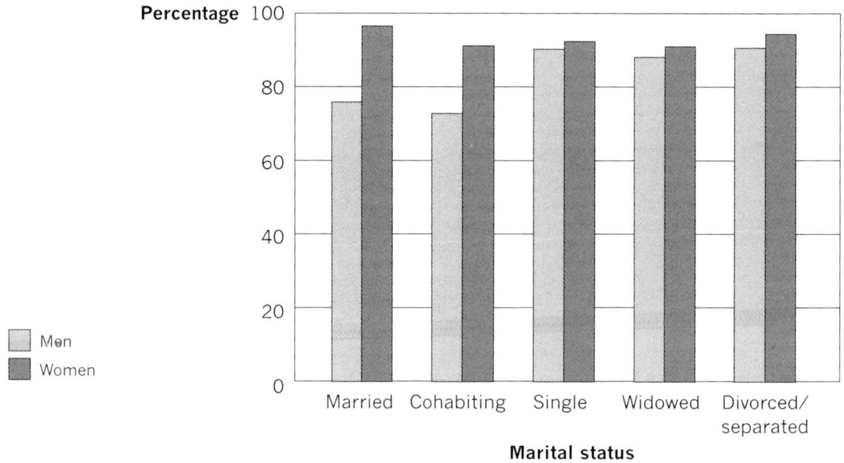

Source: Health Survey for England, 1993 and 1994

Fig. 5.7. Domestic work: percentage doing any in past four weeks by marital status: men and women aged 55+

The effect of marital status on men's and women's housework is shown in Figure 5.7. As expected, there was a significant gender difference in the proportion doing any housework only among those who were married or cohabiting. Almost all married women did some housework but only three-quarters of married men. The gender convergence in domestic work with advancing age noted above reflects the rise with age in the proportion of men and women who were widowed. About 10% of those who had no partner (widowed, single or divorced/separated) did no housework at all, suggesting that they were disabled and received informal care from relatives or from other sources.

Gardening and DIY

Like housework, these encompass a wide range of activities requiring varying amounts of physical effort. 'Light' gardening in the HSE classification includes such tasks as weeding, hoeing, pruning, planting and power-mowing, while 'light' DIY includes interior decorating, minor repairs and the washing, polishing, repairs and maintenance of a car. 'Heavy' work, which is thought to entail an intensity of effort sufficient to benefit health, includes digging, building, mowing with a push-mower, felling trees, mixing and laying concrete, moving heavy loads and refitting kitchens and bathrooms.

Figure 5.8 shows the frequency and intensity of gardening/DIY in the past four weeks for men and women by age group. Doing light gardening/DIY was common among both men and women, with over a third of all men and over a third of women under age 75 doing light

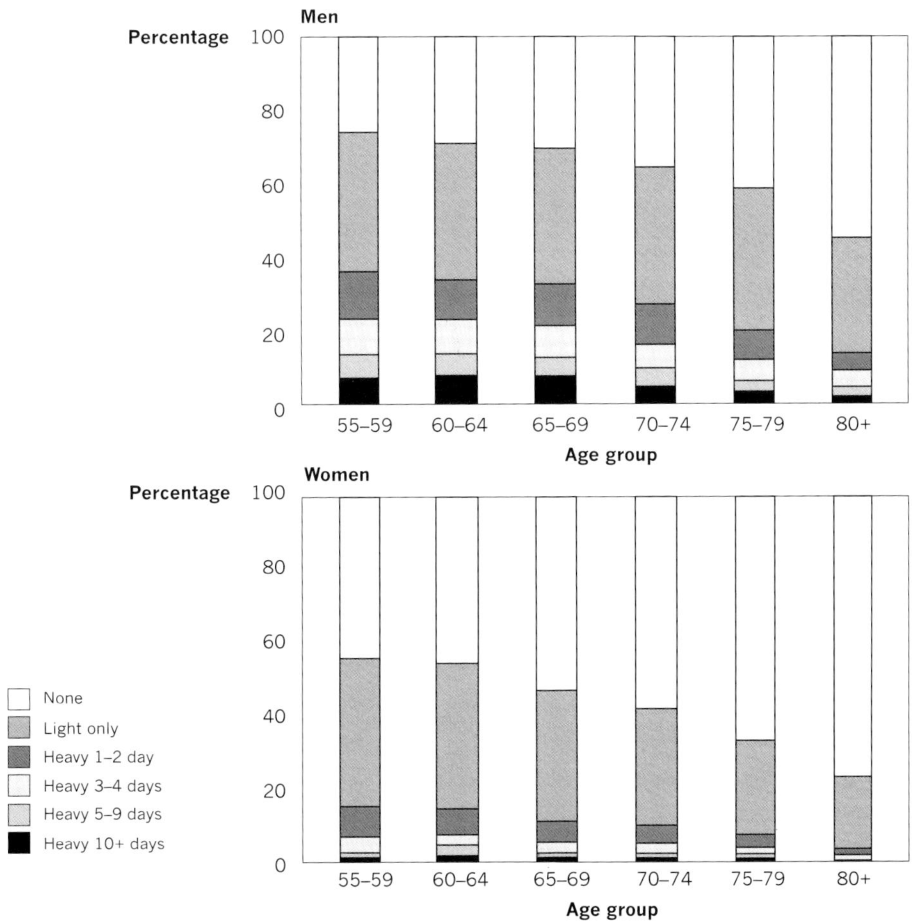

Source: Health Survey for England, 1993 and 1994

Fig. 5.8. Gardening/DIY: frequency in past four weeks and intensity by gender and age group

tasks but no heavy work. As expected, women were less likely than men to do heavy work. Thus among men aged 55–59, three-quarters did some gardening/DIY, 37% did heavy work and 7% did heavy work at least ten times in the previous four weeks. Among women in this age group the corresponding proportions were 55%, 15% and 1%. Among both men and women, the proportion doing any gardening/DIY declined with age, although for men the decline was negligible until age 70 and represented mainly a decrease in the proportion doing heavy work; for women the decline in gardening/DIY is evident from age 65 and includes a decrease in light as well as heavy work.

Men's greater participation in gardening/DIY, relative to women's, was maintained across all marital statuses, although the gender difference was most marked among those who were married or cohabiting

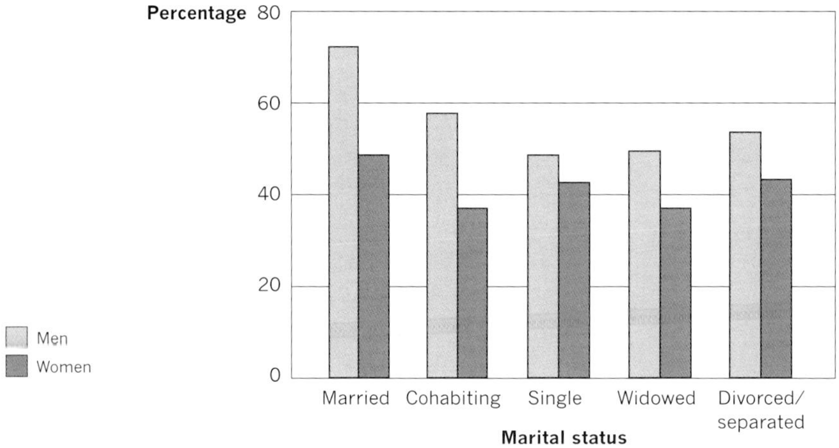

Source: Health Survey for England, 1993 and 1994

Fig. 5.9. Gardening/DIY: percentage doing any in past four weeks by marital status: men and women aged 55+

(see Figure 5.9). Whereas marital status had little effect on the overall proportion of older people doing any housework (see Figure 5.7), gardening/DIY was more common among married than non-married people.

Total physical activity

It is useful to estimate the total activity of individuals, since it is the combined effect of all physical activities which is relevant to health. The HSE provides a variable summarising the level of activity – whether none, light, moderate or vigorous – in all the activities considered, as well as in paid employment. Moderate or vigorous activity represents the intensity expected to improve health, although, as noted above, the intensity of activity required to improve the health of older people may be rather less than for younger age groups and less for women than for men. A second variable summarises both intensity and frequency of participation in any type of activity in the preceding four weeks (see Appendix C).

Figure 5.10 shows the activity (intensity and frequency) of men and women by age group. Those who did not participate in any activity or only in light activities are referred to here as 'sedentary'. Sedentariness increased among men from 22% at age 55–59 to 58% among those aged over 80; for women, the increase across the age range was steeper, from 16% to 70%. Moreover, the proportion of women whose activity was moderate or vigorous at least 12 times in the previous four weeks declined at an earlier age than men's. Thus 40% of both men and women were in this category at age 55–59, but the proportion for

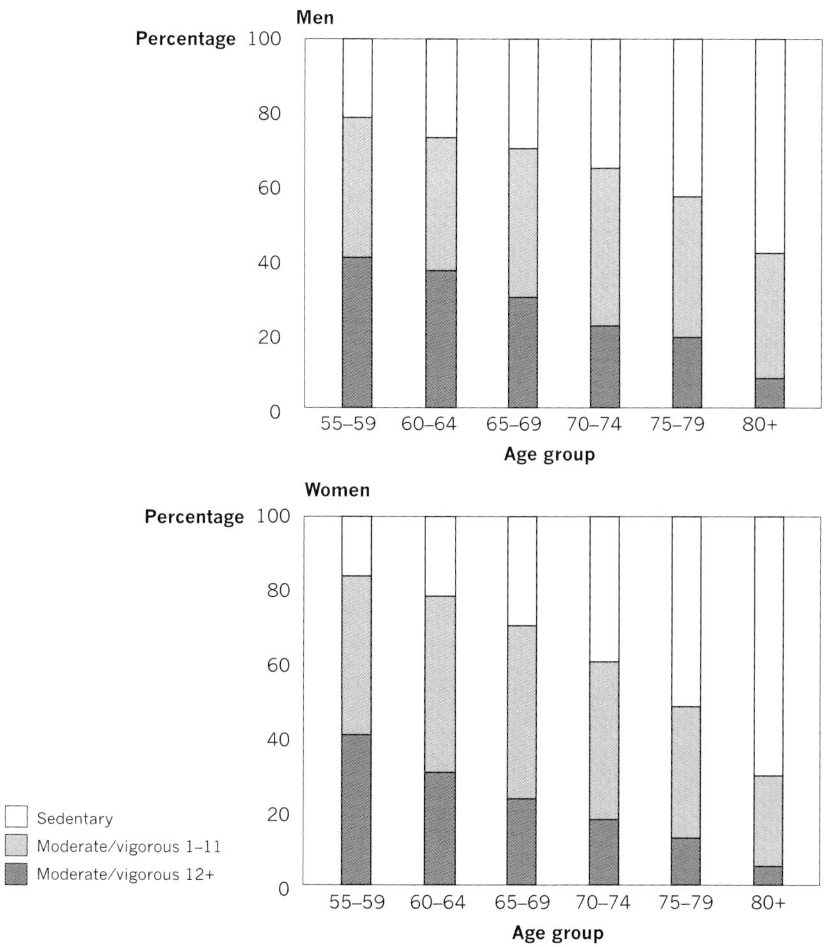

Source: Health Survey for England, 1993 and 1994

Fig. 5.10. Total activity (intensity and frequency) in past four weeks by gender and age group, aged 55+

women fell to 30% at age 60–64, whereas the proportion of men did not fall to this level until age 65–69. In sum, the gender gap in activity level and frequency widened with age.

Having described the participation rates of men and women in four kinds of physical activities – recreational, walking, domestic and gardening/DIY – and in activities as a whole, we now consider possible explanations for the low levels of participation and for the decline with age, in terms of health constraints, cultural norms and material constraints.

Effects of health, material resources, educational level and social class on physical activity

Health

Barriers to older people's participation in activities may include both physical limitations and a lack of confidence in the ability to manage physical activities safely. Self-efficacy – 'a judgement of one's capability to accomplish a certain level of performance' (Bandura, 1986, p. 391) – has been shown to be important in explaining willingness to adopt a regular exercise routine among adults (Sallis *et al.*, 1992; Marcus and Owen, 1992). This is echoed in the qualitative research by Finch (1997) on older people, which revealed a fear of health risks from physical exertion and uncertainty as to safe levels of exercise.

Disabilities and disease conditions which develop with advancing age are therefore likely to have a double impact on physical activity. Practical difficulties, such as pain on movement, loss of balance, impaired muscular control and breathlessness, affect physical capabilitities directly but also reduce the individual's confidence in engaging in physical exercise (Clark, 1996). We would expect that the level and frequency of physical activity are strongly associated with health.

Although the HSE records long-standing illness, there is no measure of functional disability or of limitations on activity associated with long-standing illness; these must be inferred from their contribution to self-assessed health, which is recorded as very good, good, fair, bad or very bad. Figure 5.11 shows that the proportion of men and women whose physical activity in the previous four weeks had reached at least a moderate intensity was closely related to their self-assessed health; among men who reported their health as 'very good' or 'good', 80% had engaged in moderate or vigorous activity, compared with only 15% among those who said their health was 'very bad'. The pattern for women was very similar, indicating that gender differences in activity levels are at least partly explained by gender differences in self-assessed health.

Figure 5.12 shows the level and frequency of men's and women's physical activity by age group and by self-assessed health, grouped into three categories. The effect of health is greater than that of age; for example, among men in the youngest age group (55–59) sedentariness ranged from 12%, where health was good, to 64%, where it was bad, whereas in the oldest age group (over 80) only 46% of men in good health were sedentary. However, advancing age was still associated with a lower level and frequency of activity after controlling for self-assessed health. The greater effect of age on women's than men's activity (see

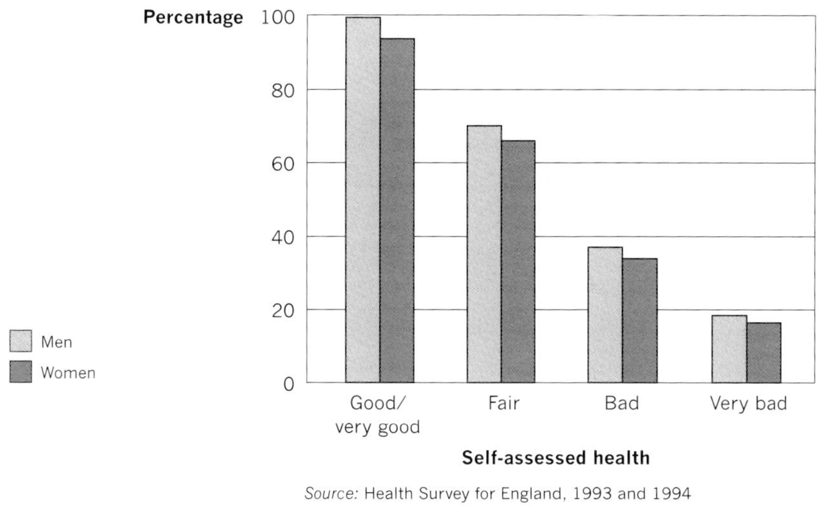

Fig. 5.11. Percentage of men and women who were active at a moderate or vigorous level, by self-assessed health

Figure 5.10) was somewhat reduced after taking account of health. Thus poor health places more severe limits on activity than age *per se*.

Social class, material resources and education

Older people's view of appropriate and manageable physical activity may be related to their social class background. Clark (1996) argues that exercise self-efficacy, or confidence in physical capability, develops mainly through successful experiences of activity (Clark, Patrick, Grembowski and Durham, 1995; McAuley, Lox and Duncan, 1993). It is also influenced by observing others as role models, including family, peers and examples presented in the media, and through verbal encouragement by health care professionals, family and the media. Participation in recreational activities is therefore likely to reflect preferences for leisure pursuits developed earlier in the life course, which may be cohort-specific and also influenced by class-related opportunities and friendship networks. Changing exercise habits in mid-life or later life may be difficult, especially where friends in the same age group are sedentary. For example, qualitative research has shown that recreational activity is inhibited by a reluctance to do something new and unaccustomed as well as diffidence in going to a class or club alone (Finch, 1997). Lack of companions will be more likely where an activity is uncommon or perceived as inappropriate among one's age group or social class.

Moreover, as Clark (1996) argues, socioeconomic status (including occupational class, education and income) affects an individual's sense

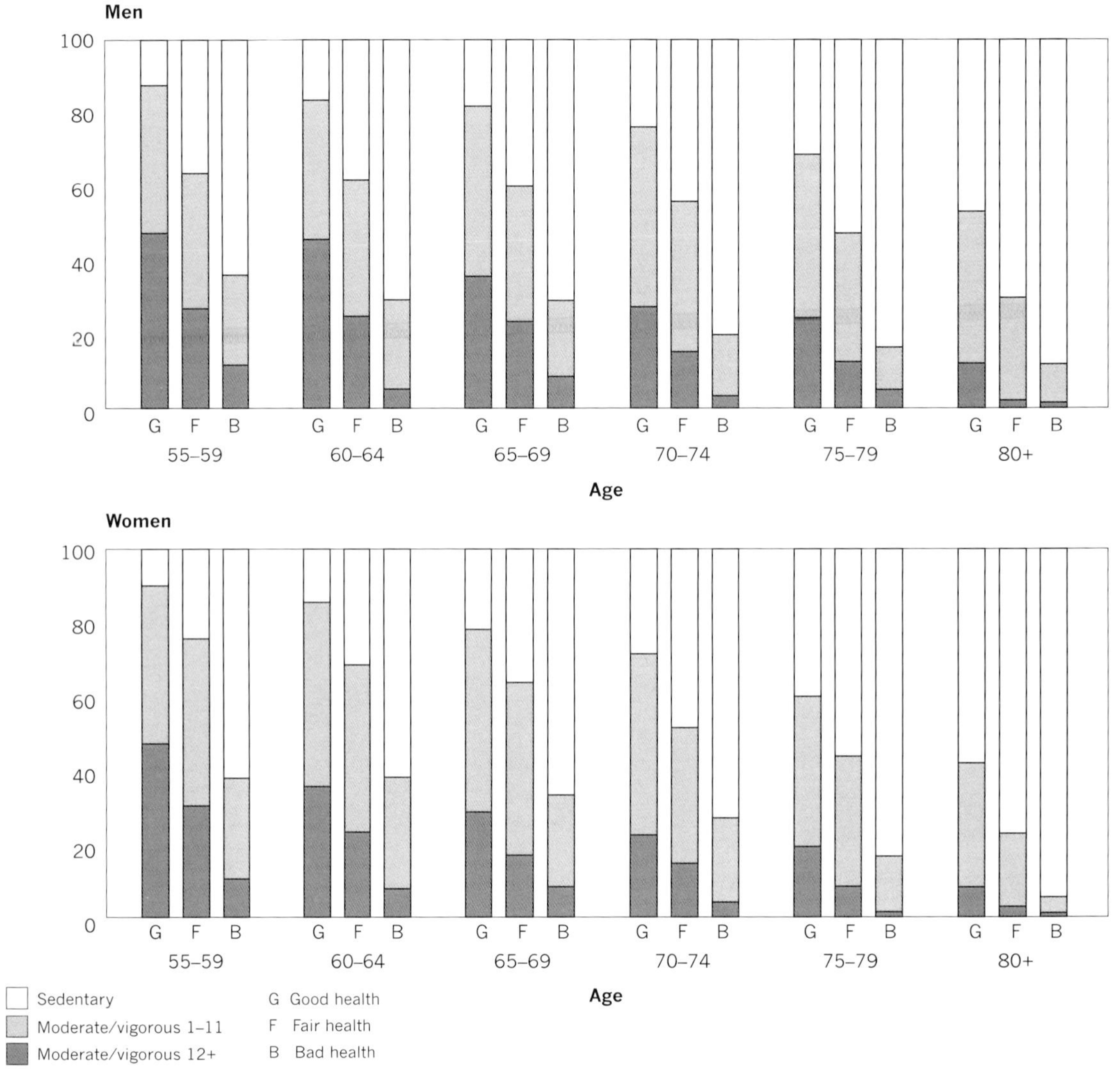

Source: Health Survey for England, 1993 and 1994

Fig. 5.12. Total activity (intensity and frequency) by self-assessed health, age group and gender, aged 55+

of control, or ability to cope with challenges in their life. Fatalism, or lack of a sense of control of one's health, is more common among older people in lower occupational classes (see Chapter 2). We use socioeconomic group, based on each individual's current or last main occupation and grouped into six categories (SECs), as a measure of class. A seventh category represents those (mainly women) who had never been employed (see Appendix A for further details).

Some recreational activities were clearly associated with class but others were not. For example, a greater proportion swam in the higher

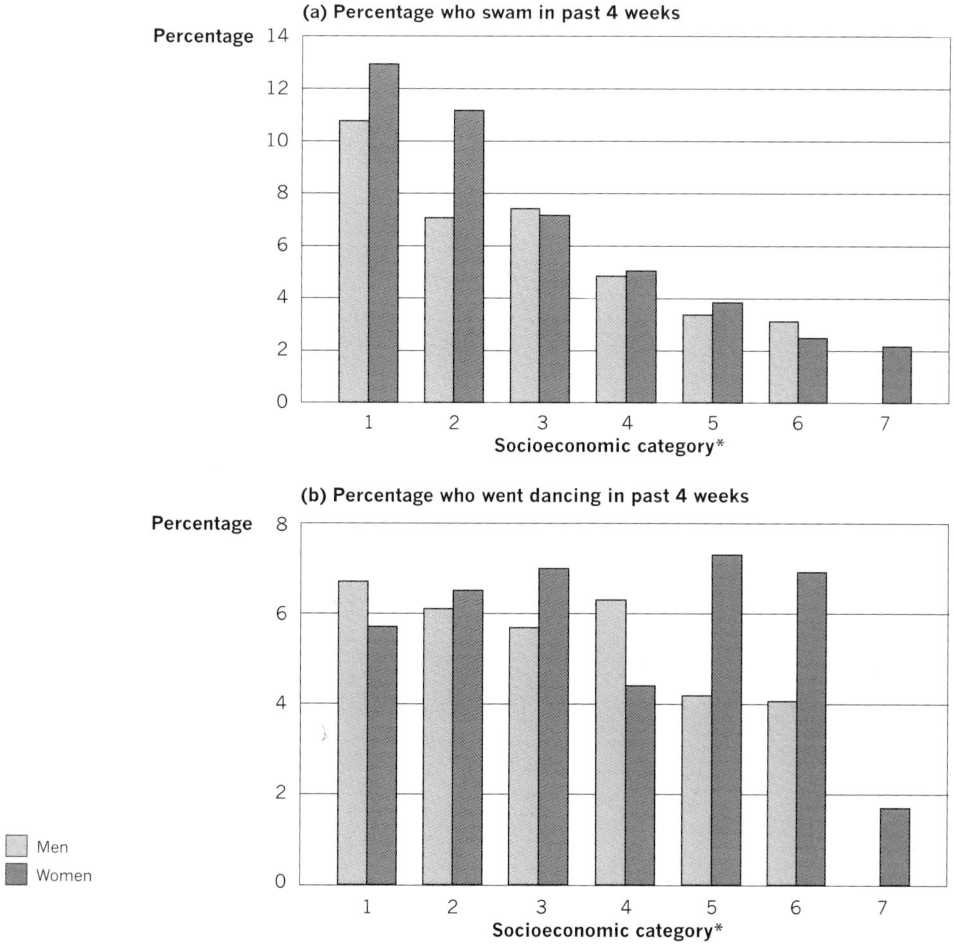

* See Appendix A

Source: Health Survey for England, 1993 and 1994

Fig. 5.13. Recreational activities by social class of men and women aged 55+

than the lower socioeconomic groups, 13% of women and nearly 11% of men in SEC 1 (professionals, managers in large organisations and employers) compared with less than 3% in SEC 6 (unskilled manual) (see Figure 5.13(a)). The class gradient in swimming was stronger for women than for men. In contrast, there was no clear relationship between dancing and social class (see Figure 5.13(b)). Women in the semi-skilled and unskilled groups (SEC 5 and 6) were slightly more likely to have been dancing than women in SEC 1 but the reverse was the case for men.

Some activities require payment of membership or entry fees; in addition, club and facilities may be too far away to reach on foot, so that the cost of travelling, either by bus or car, adds to the expense.

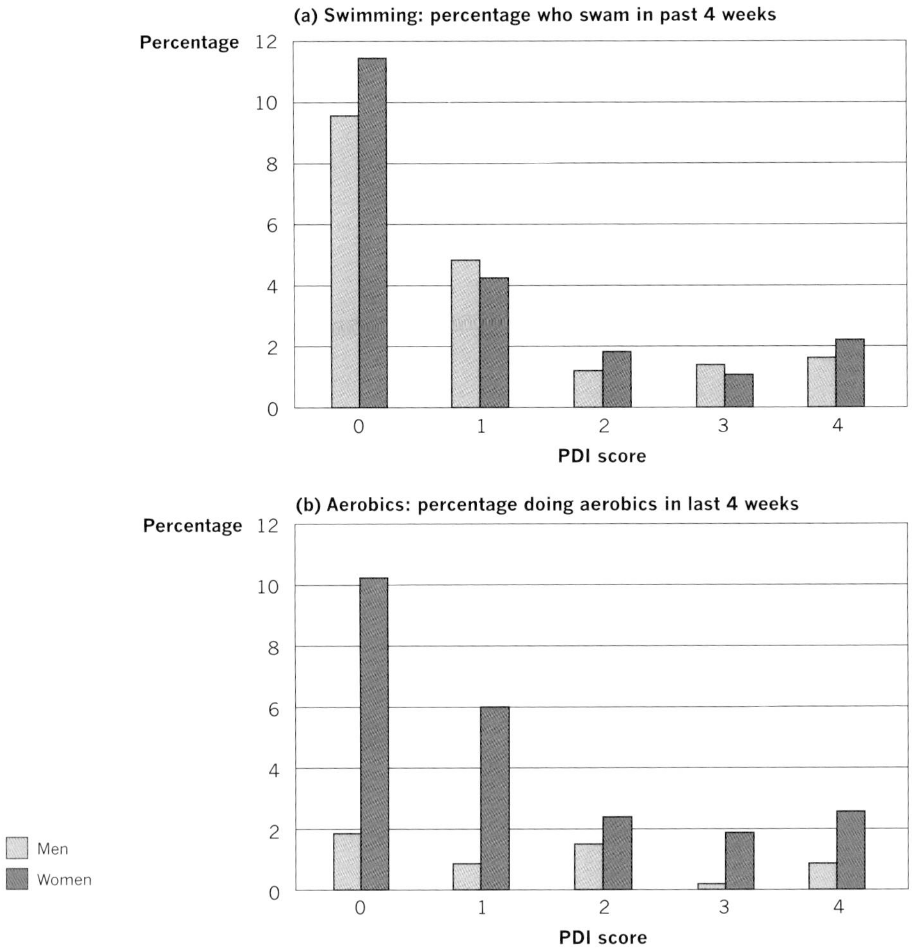

Source: Health Survey for England, 1993 and 1994

Fig. 5.14. Recreational activities by personal deprivation index (PDI) of men and women aged 55+

Where an activity takes place in the evening, women in particular may be reluctant to attend unless they can travel by car, owing to a common perception that the streets are unsafe at night. Even walking is often more difficult for the urban poor, due to noisy and polluted streets, uneven pavements, greater crime and fear of crime. Thus material deprivation and security concerns may deter physical exercise. As the HSE provides no information about income, we have constructed a measure of personal deprivation, with a score of 0–4 based on housing tenure, access to a car and telephone, having central heating in the household, whether unemployed and whether reliant on Income Support (see Appendix A for details).

In Figure 5.14 the relationship between personal deprivation score

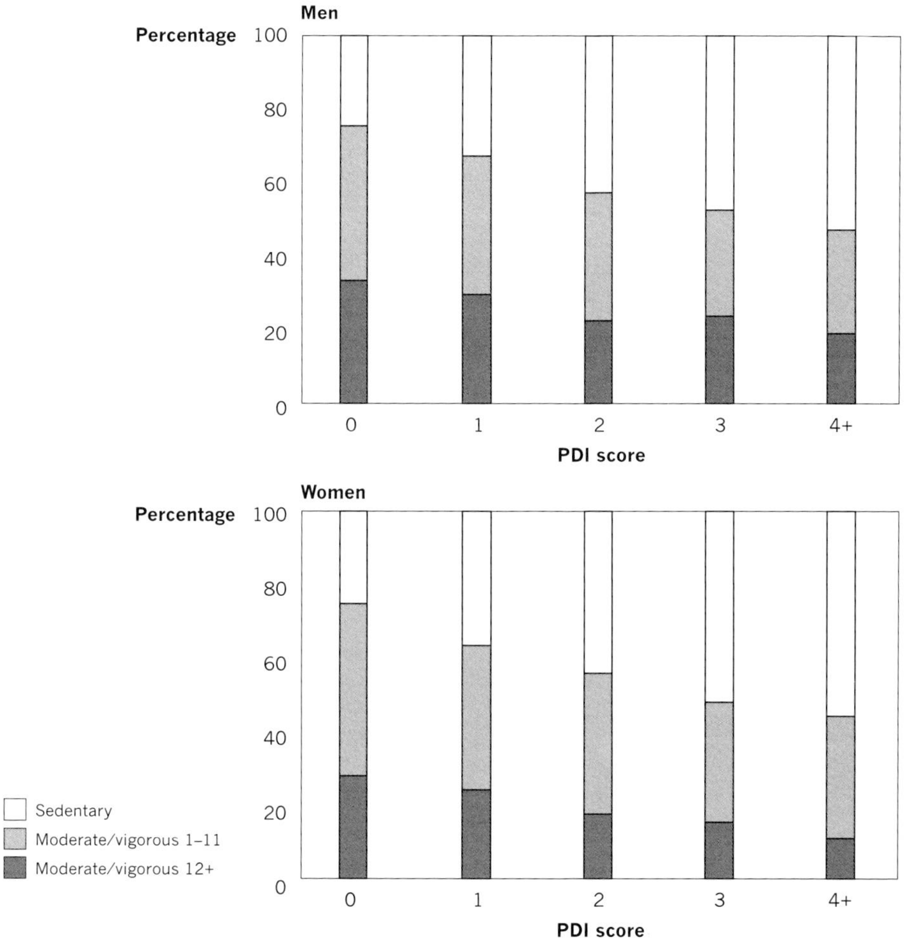

Source: Health Survey for England, 1993 and 1994

Fig. 5.15. Total activity (intensity and frequency): men and women aged 55+ by personal deprivation index (PDI)

and two illustrative activities, swimming (a) and aerobics (b) is shown. Swimming declined sharply from the most advantaged group (score 0) to the middle group (score 3), with low levels maintained for men and women in the most deprived groups. Aerobics followed a similar pattern for women. These associations, which are also evident for the other recreational activities, are consistent with the hypothesis that material deprivation exerts a constraint on such activities.

Total physical activity also declined with increasing deprivation (see Figure 5.15). The proportions who were sedentary, with an activity level not reaching a moderate intensity, was a quarter among men and women in the most advantaged group (with a personal deprivation score of 0) but increased to over 40% for the middle group (score 2)

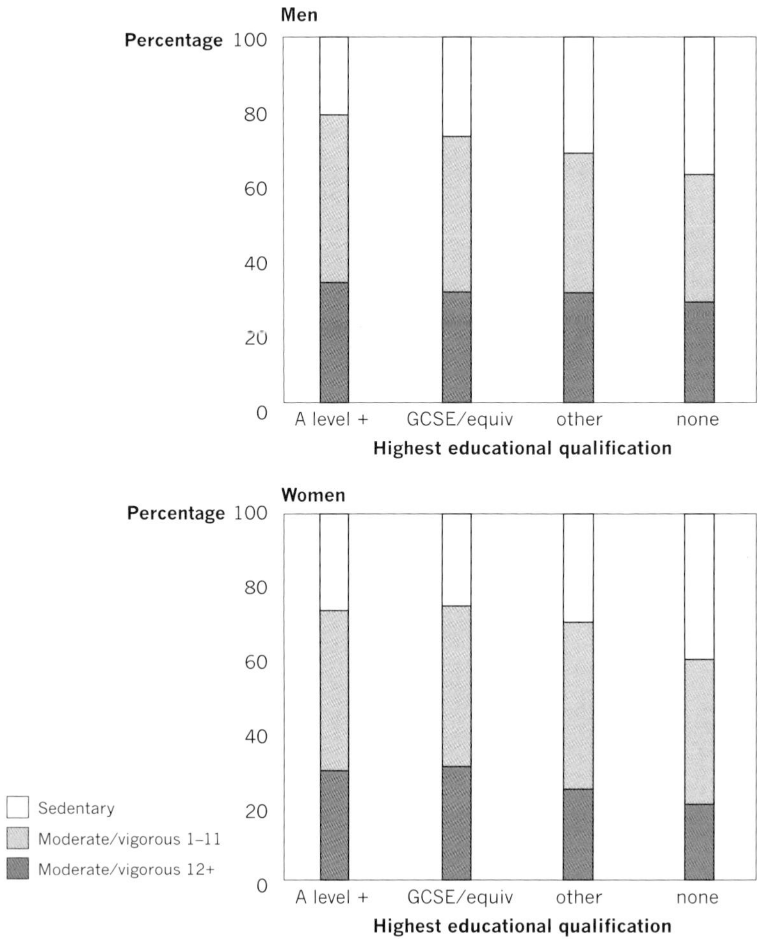

Source: Health Survey for England, 1993 and 1994

Fig. 5.16. Total activity (intensity and frequency): men and women aged 55+ by educational qualifications

and reached over half among the most materially deprived group (score of 4 or more). Women were slightly more likely than men to be sedentary within each group and substantially less likely to engage in moderate or vigorous activity at least 12 times in the previous four weeks. The strong association between inactivity and deprivation is likely to reflect the constraints discussed above.

Education, it has been suggested, enhances the adoption and maintenance of a healthy lifestyle (Williams, 1990). Education provides the opportunity to engage in less hazardous occupations (Leigh, 1983); educated individuals also have a greater awareness of health risks and are more receptive to health advice, being less inclined to a fatalistic view (Fuchs, 1979; Grossman, 1976). Thus those who are more highly educated may be more responsive to health promotion messages concerning the value to health of physical exercise. Among older people, many ceased full-time education before reaching age 16 and about half of those aged over 55 reported no educational qualifications. Figure 5.16 shows some decline in total activity with decreasing educational level. For example, among those lacking any qualifications, nearly 40% were sedentary, compared with under 25% among those whose highest qualification was at least A level or equivalent.

The lower participation rates of the materially deprived in recreational activities and in overall activity may be partly due to the fact that the most disadvantaged tend also to be older and to have a higher prevalence of chronic disability and illness, both of which would limit physical activity. Multivariate analysis is necessary to disentangle the separate effects of age, ill health, gender, marital status, social class, educational level and material deprivation on physical activity levels.

Multivariate analysis

Logistic regression analysis was used to estimate the odds of being sedentary, that is, having taken part in no physical activity or only light activity in the previous four weeks. The proportion of respondents who were sedentary was 32% of men and 36% of women.

Tables 5.1 and 5.2 show the odds ratios of being sedentary for men and women over age 55. In Model 1, only age group was included and in Model 2 variables for self-assessed health and chronic illness were added. For men, including educational level and the Personal Deprivation Index (PDI) improved the fit of the model. For women the effect of educational level was not statistically significant but the effect of socioeconomic category was (and is included in Table 5.2). Marital status had no significant effect on activity levels and was therefore omitted from the models.

For both men and women, advancing age was strongly associated with declining activity, even after controlling for health, but the effect of age was much greater for women than for men. For example, the odds of sedentariness were nearly 13 times greater for women aged over 80 compared with those aged 55–59 (the reference category) (see Model 1 for women); the corresponding odds ratio for men was 5.06. Men had a ten-year advantage over women in terms of the rate of decline in activity with age; women's odds of sedentariness, relative to the odds at age 55–59, were doubled by age 65–69, whereas for men, the odds were not doubled until age 75–79. This gender difference was maintained after other variables were added to the model.

Having a longstanding illness increased the odds of sedentariness for

Table 5.1. Odds ratios of being sedentary for men aged 55+ years

	Model 1	Model 2	Model 3	Model 4
Age	†††	†††	†††	†††
55–59	1.00	1.00	1.00	1.00
60–64	1.36 **	1.32 *	1.29 *	1.29 *
65–69	1.57 ***	1.41 **	1.35 **	1.36 **
70–74	2.07 ***	1.92 ***	1.82 ***	1.82 ***
75–79	2.81 ***	2.67 ***	2.55 ***	2.46 ***
80+	5.06 ***	5.12 ***	4.81 ***	4.55 ***
Chronic health status		†††	†††	†††
No long-standing illness		1.00	1.00	1.00
Long-standing illness		1.32 ***	1.35	1.37 ***
General health		†††	†††	†††
Very good/good		1.00	1.00	1.00
Fair		2.62 ***	2.48 ***	2.40 ***
Bad		7.97 ***	7.49 ***	6.85 ***
Very bad		18.89 ***	17.13 ***	15.74 ***
Highest educational qualifications			†††	†
A-level or above			1.00	1.00
O-level or equivalent			1.21	1.18
Other			1.30 *	1.21
None			1.50 ***	1.35 **
PDI				†††
0				1.00
1				1.07
2				1.28 *
3				1.41 *
4+				2.03 ***
Δ –2LLR	218	597	17	22
Δ df	5	4	3	4
N =	4673			

Statistical significance of variable in the model; † $P < 0.05$; †† $P < 0.01$; ††† $P < 0.001$.
Statistical significance of difference from reference category, * $P < 0.05$; ** $P < 0.01$; *** $P < 0.001$.
Source: Health Survey for England, 1993 and 1994

Table 5.2. Odds ratios of being sedentary for women aged 55+ years

	Model 1	Model 2	Model 3	Model 4
Age	†††	†††	†††	†††
55–59	1.00	1.00	1.00	1.00
60–64	1.48 ***	1.53 ***	1.52 ***	1.51 ***
65–69	2.25 ***	2.20 ***	2.16 ***	2.16 ***
70–74	3.45 ***	3.31 ***	3.17 ***	3.13 ***
75–79	5.94 ***	5.35 ***	5.04 ***	4.95 ***
80+	12.87 ***	12.25 ***	11.23 ***	10.88 ***
Chronic health status		†††	†††	†††
No longstanding illness		1.00	1.00	1.00
Longstanding illness		1.45 ***	1.46 ***	1.46 ***
General health		†††	†††	†††
Very good/good		1.00	1.00	1.00
Fair		2.09 ***	2.03 ***	2.03 ***
Bad		6.47 ***	6.11 ***	6.04 ***
Very bad		13.63 ***	12.73 ***	12.59 ***
Highest educational qualifications			ns	ns
PDI			†††	†††
0			1.00	1.00
1			1.15	1.17
2			1.12	1.13
3			1.25 *	1.28 *
4+			1.85 ***	1.92 ***
Socioeconomic category				†††
Professionals/large managers				1.00
Intermediate non-manual/small managers				0.74
Routine non-manual				0.75
Skilled manual				0.68 *
Semi-skilled				0.77
Unskilled manual				0.77
Never worked				1.53
Δ –2LLR	850	547	19	24
Δ df	5	4	4	6
N =	5958			

Statistical significance of variable in the model: † $P < 0.05$; †† $P < 0.01$; ††† $P < 0.001$.
Statistical significance of difference from reference category: * $P < 0.05$; ** $P < 0.01$; *** $P < 0.001$.

Source: Health Survey for England, 1993 and 1994

both men and women, but the effect of self-assessed health was much greater (see Model 2). Poor self-assessed health was the most important constraint on activity of both men and women. Thus for men whose health was only 'fair', the odds of sedentariness were over twice that of men reporting 'very good' or 'good' health; for men with 'very bad' health, the odds ratio was nearly 19.

For men, those with no educational qualifications had raised odds of sedentariness 1.5 times the odds of those with the highest qualifications.

Material resources, as measured by the PDI, had a significant effect on the likelihood of sedentariness for both men and women (see Model 4 for men, Model 3 for women). The most disadvantaged men, with a PDI of 4 or more, had odds over twice that of the most advantaged, whose PDI was 0. The effect of deprivation on women's activity was slightly less, mainly because class was also included in Model 4 for women.

Class had no effect for men on 'sedentariness' but did for women. Perhaps surprisingly, women who had been professionals or employers or managers in large organisations were more likely to be sedentary than those in the skilled manual group. There is some indication that women who had never been employed, who may have had some long-term disabling condition, were more likely to be sedentary than the professional group, although this result fell short of statistical significance.

The effects of self-assessed health and of age were somewhat reduced by adding material resources to Model 3 for men; the odds ratio of sedentariness was reduced from 4.81 to 4.55 for those aged over 80 and from 17.13 to 15.74 for those reporting very bad health. For women, adding material resources and class to Model 2 also reduced the effects of age and health. Thus the association of material deprivation with sedentariness is partly due to the fact that material deprivation is associated with older age and poorer health.

Discussion and conclusions

This chapter has described older people's participation in various kinds of physical activity, including recreational exercise, domestic work, gardening/DIY and walking over the previous four weeks. Variation according to age, gender, health, marital status, social class and material resources was analysed.

The decline in physical activity with age was far more pronounced for women than men, the latter showing a relatively stable level of activity until age 70. Men's decline in total physical activity occurred at a later age than women's and was more closely linked to poor self-assessed health.

Domestic and gardening/DIY activity highlighted the gendered division of labour, with women performing the bulk of domestic work and men more likely to work in the garden or on DIY tasks. Gender convergence with advancing age was evident in domestic work, because of women's steeper decline in domestic activity with age. The gender division of tasks around the home was, as expected, most evident among those who were married or cohabiting, although marital status had no effect on the level of physical activity as a whole.

Participation in physical recreation of any kind other than walking was about a third for men and a quarter for women, although each of the four most popular activities (swimming, cycling, dancing and exercises) attracted only 5–10% of older people. Aerobics was a less common activity and dominated by women, whereas cycling was dominated by men. The proportion doing exercises, including sit-ups and press-ups, showed less decline with age than other activities. Marital status had a significant effect only on dancing, where single (never married) people were less likely to have been dancing than other people. Most physical recreational activities were less common among those who were materially deprived or in a low social class, suggesting that lack of financial resources or private transport constrain participation in such activities.

Walking was, as expected, much more common than physical recreational activities. Of those aged 55–59, 60% had taken walks of at least a mile in the previous four weeks, and even in their late 70s over half of men and 40% of women had done so. However, few walked at a brisk pace, so that the direct physiological benefits may have been rather limited.

Health itself was the most important predictor of physical activity, outweighing the effect of age; those who assessed their own health as poor were far less likely to be active at a moderate level, within each age group. As well as placing physical limitations on activity, poor health may also influence older people's exercise self-efficacy, reducing their confidence in their ability to perform activities successfully and exacerbating fears of the health risks involved.

Older people are more vulnerable than younger to being caught in a vicious cycle, or downward spiral, of health impairment, reduced physical activity and further decline in fitness, health and wellbeing. In so far as negative attitudes towards exercise contribute to this process, intervention needs to focus on reassurance and practical suggestions from health professionals as to ways in which older people can exercise safely, taking into account their particular limitations. Successful experiences of physical activity, which enhance wellbeing and a sense of control, especially where shared with peers, should tend to encourage positive attitudes to exercise, gradually building both confidence and physical capacity. For men, there is some evidence of education having a positive association with physical activity.

However, adopting a healthier exercise routine is not merely a matter of changing attitudes. Although social class had little effect on physical activity level after taking account of health and age, lack of material resources was strongly associated with sedentariness, which was more likely among those who were materially deprived, after controlling for health and age; the most deprived older people had double the odds of a sedentary lifestyle compared with the most advantaged. This may reflect multiple barriers to physical activity, including the costs of participating in recreational activities and of transport, cramped accommodation and lack of a garden. The most deprived older people are also more likely to live in a neighbourhood unsuitable for walking, in terms of both the built and the social environment.

The promotion of physical activity among older people needs to take account of the constraints on participation arising from both deprived material circumstances and from poor health. A range of attractive, low-cost, locally accessible or home-based physical activities needs to be available for older people, in which even those in poor health can participate safely.

6 Social and structural factors associated with diet and smoking

Introduction

In this chapter, we examine the influence of structural factors and social circumstances on two aspects of older people's health-related behaviour – diet and smoking. Among the social circumstances considered are social support, marital status, living arrangements and psychosocial health; structural factors are indicated by past occupational class and by an index of material deprivation. Diet and smoking both have well-established and significant effects on health and mortality, whereas it is not so clear that alcohol consumed in moderate amounts is damaging to health (Doll, 1997, and see Chapter 4). By analysing diet and smoking, we show how far there is a common pattern of variation in health-related behaviour or whether patterns differ depending on which aspect is considered.

In seeking explanations for the link between health inequalities and class, debate has focused on whether health is mainly influenced by the structural/material conditions in which people live or by cultural/behavioural factors (Blane, 1985; Macintyre, 1986; Townsend, Davidson and Whitehead, 1988). Proponents of the cultural/behavioural explanation have emphasised personal responsibility for health behaviour, playing down any constraints arising from social background and from current material and social circumstances.

Others have rejected an individualistic interpretation of health behaviour as blaming the disadvantaged for their poorer health (Nettleton, 1996) and have argued that health behaviour is influenced both by material circumstances and by cultural norms which operate at the level of society and within class and ethnic groupings. Thus: 'what is attributed to individual choice is in fact substantially shaped by powerful economic and social forces, the goods and facilities that are immediately available and level of income' (Townsend, Phillimore and Beattie, 1988, p. xiv). In this interpretation, with which we concur, health-related behaviour is likely to be influenced by the material conditions in which a person lives, by their social class, by gender and possibly also by a range of social circumstances, including social support, marital status, living arrangements and stress. Although this range of social circumstances has been analysed for their impact on health, studies which consider their role in promoting healthy behaviour are less common. A key concern is therefore to assess the relative importance of social circumstances to older people's health behaviour compared with the influence of class and material resources.

We first outline recent survey evidence on variations in the diet of individuals aged over 55, before reviewing the ways in which class, material resources and social circumstances may influence this aspect of personal lifestyle. A review of evidence on older people's smoking has already been provided in Chapter 3. The next section outlines our data and methods, while the main part of the chapter presents our analysis.

Variation in diet among older people

Consumption of a variety of items was compared in the HSE according to age group, gender and social class of the head of household (Colhoun and Prescott-Clarke, 1996, tables 7.6–7.18). Those aged over 65 were slightly more likely than younger people to eat white rather than other bread and less likely to use skimmed milk, but for other items their diet was at least as healthy as for younger people.

Among those aged over 65, women and those in higher social classes had more healthy eating habits than men and those in lower social classes. For example, 46% of men aged over 65 used sugar in tea compared with 26% of women; 61% of men in classes IV and V used sugar compared with 34% of men in classes I and II. A similar pattern was evident for use of sugar in coffee, white rather than brown or wholemeal bread, whole rather than skimmed milk, infrequent consumption of fruit, vegetables or high-fibre cereals, routinely adding salt at table and not taking vitamin supplements. In sum, diets are more healthy among older women than men and among those in non-manual occupational groups.

This finding is consistent with research in the US on people of all age groups (Ginn, Arber and Cooper, 1997). Using data from the Continuing Survey of Food Intakes of Individuals, a Healthy Eating Index, based on ten dietary components and reflecting conformity to the Dietary Guidelines for Americans and the Food Guide Pyramid, was constructed. Women had healthier diets than men and individuals living in jointly headed or female-headed households had better diets than those in male-headed households. Diets were better for those with higher levels of education and, to a lesser extent, for those with higher incomes.

To summarise, the lifestyle of people aged over 65 is not less healthy than that of younger people. As shown in Chapter 3, current smoking is less common and, as discussed above, diet is not markedly poorer. Older people's capacity to improve their health behaviour is shown in the proportion of smokers who quit; a substantial proportion of people aged over 60 in 1984/5 had given up smoking in the interval between the two Health and Lifestyle Surveys, 13% of men and 9% of women (Whichelow and Cox, 1993).

Factors affecting health behaviour

Class and material resources

It is important to measure the independent effects of both class and current material resources on health behaviours since these cannot be assumed to have the same effect. The 'class approach' to health inequalities, exemplified by the Black Report (Department of Health and Social Security, 1980), was mainly concerned with men of working age, while the 'poverty approach', measuring access to material resources, analyses mortality of both men and women of working age (e.g. Fox and Goldblatt, 1982). Although older people have been relatively neglected in both approaches, recent research has shown that previous occupational class continues to be an important predictor of morbidity in later life, and that health differentials among older people are also associated with current material resources (Arber and Ginn, 1991, 1993; Arber and Cooper, 1999).

The work of Townsend and colleagues (Townsend, Davidson and Whitehead, 1988; Townsend, Phillimore and Beattie, 1988) bridges the two traditions, examining the effects of poor housing, lack of a car and low income, as well as of low social class and area of residence, on health behaviour:

> smoking and eating habits ... are far from activities determined solely by individual choice. Diet is profoundly influenced by cultural or local social customs, informal and formal education, the availability as well as price of goods in local markets (Townsend, Phillimore and Beattie, 1988, p. xiv).

Research has suggested that social circumstances, such as social support, marriage, living with others, close friendship and religious affiliation, are beneficial to health. But the question of whether or how these factors influence people's health-related behaviour is not well understood, especially for older people.

Social support

Social support has been recognised as a valuable resource for maintaining health and lowering mortality (Berkman and Syme, 1979; Cohen and Syme, 1985), although two aspects of social support – the perceived emotional quality of a person's relationships and the amount and frequency of social contact – may influence health in different ways (Qureshi, 1990). Several hypotheses have been proposed to explain how social support contributes to health (see Cooper *et al.*, 1999). The first is that social support acts as a buffer against the stresses of life, protecting the individual from the pathogenic effects of stress on health (Cohen and Willis, 1985; World Health Organisation, 1992; Bankoff, 1983). The second is that social support improves health directly through the beneficial effects of enhanced self-esteem and sense of security (Thoits, 1982). A third explanation is that health behaviour is influenced by close relationships and social networks (Abella and Heslin, 1984; Langlie, 1977; Jerrome, 1990). In this research, we investigate whether older people's health behaviour is related to social support, in terms of the perceived quality of close relationships.

Marital status and solo living

The greater longevity of married people has been frequently demonstrated, theorised as due to a 'health protective' effect, in which marriage increases social networks, encourages healthy behaviour, provides informal care, increases economic resources and buffers against stress. Alternatively, healthier individuals may be selected into marriage (Goldman, Korenman and Weinstein, 1995). A longitudinal study by the same authors on older people in the US found the protective effect of marriage is the more important and confirms the positive association of a socially active lifestyle with better health outcomes. Although the health of older people living alone is similar to that of other older people, this partly reflects the selection process whereby the most frail move to live with others or into residential care.

Older people are particularly vulnerable to lack of social contact associated with the death or institutionalisation of partner, siblings or members of their peer group, but women are more likely be widowed than men because of the marriage age differential and women's greater longevity. Thus nearly half of older women are widows (47%), most of whom live alone, compared with only 17% of men (Office for National Statistics, 1997, calculated from table 7).

The impact of widowhood is likely to differ between men and women for several reasons (Arber and Ginn, 1991; Davidson, 1998). For married men, their wife is often their only confidante, whereas a close friend is more likely to perform this role for married women. Widowhood may affect men's diet more than women's, owing to women's traditional role in selecting, preparing and cooking food; men may therefore, at least initially, suffer a deterioration in their diet when widowed. Widows may find it more difficult than widowers to maintain relationships with married friends (Lopata, 1971), while lacking the supportive social networks built up over time by single women. Living alone restricts opportunities for social interaction, especially if mobility is limited, there is no access to private transport and if public transport is infrequent or unaffordable, conditions which are more common among older women than men; older women are less likely than men to have access to a car and have lower personal income than men (Arber and Ginn, 1991). Because of the different implications of marriage, bereavement and solo living for men and women, we would expect any effects of marital status on health behaviour to interact with gender.

Stress

Psychosocial wellbeing is likely to decline with age as a result of loss of roles and attachments. The HALS of 1991/2 (Cox, Huppert and Whichelow, 1993) confirmed that among those aged over 67, high malaise, as measured by the 12-item GHQ (GHQ12), was more common among those living alone (Swain, 1993). Longitudinal analysis showed that psychosocial health declined over a seven-year interval among those aged over 65, especially among men who had retired early and among those who had become widowed (Huppert and Whittington, 1993). The HALS shows that stress among men and women aged over 65, as indicated by the GHQ12 score, was raised among those whose level of perceived social support was very low and also among those with acute or long-standing illness (Cox, Huppert and Whichelow, 1993, table 3.18).

It has been suggested that stress – whether from illness, from loss of social interaction and support, from adverse life events or from living in materially deprived living conditions – may lead to health-damaging behaviour (Marsh and McKay, 1994). For example, among young mothers who smoke, the psychosocial benefits of smoking – including stress release – are perceived as outweighing the health-damaging effects, which they are aware of (Graham, 1987). In a similar way, heavy drinking or comfort eating may represent a response to stress and depression. Because of this possibility, we analyse whether health behaviour is related to stress, as indicated by the GHQ12 instrument.

The main aim of this chapter is to improve understanding of what influences older people's diet and smoking. In order to assess their relative importance to health behaviour, it is necessary to analyse simultaneously the effects of structural factors (class and material resources) and the effects of social factors (marital status, living arrangements, social support and stress).

Data and methods

In nutritional research, assessment of the quality of diet is often based on a food diary, including weights of foods consumed, recorded over a specified period and compared with recommended intake of foods. The DINE system (Dennison, Dennison and Frank, 1994) represents a method of standardising and streamlining the assessment of diet quality, yet still requires more information than is available in the HSE. Nevertheless, the HSE does (in 1993 and 1994) include a series of questions on consumption of food items which allow inference to be made as to an individual's dietary habits.

Respondents were asked about the type of milk, cereals, bread and spread used, about their means of frying, use of salt, and frequency of eating bread, vegetables, fruit, pulses, cakes, sweets and biscuits. A diet index, in which a higher score represents a healthier diet, was constructed by applying the principles underlying the Healthy Diet Score of Dowler and Calvert (1995) (see Appendix D for examples of calculation of the diet index). Our diet score is an indicator rather than a measure of diet, as it is not based on information as to the quantities of all foods consumed over a period. The quality of the diet is inferred from information on the type and frequency of consumption for only a limited range of foods.

Married people were distinguished from those who were living as a couple (cohabiting) in the analysis, since the latter group is likely to differ in its social characteristics from the former, especially among older people, whose socialisation placed a stronger taboo on cohabiting than for later cohorts. However, the numbers cohabiting were small, 48 men and 35 women. Similarly, it was desirable to distinguish non-married people living alone from the minority living with others, since the latter are likely to share meals and to have limited control over their diet. Results based on all these small groups must be regarded as tentative.

Psychosocial health or stress was measured by the GHQ12, a self-completion screening instrument designed to detect psychiatric disorders in the general population (Goldberg, 1972). The items include concentration, lost sleep, feelings of usefulness, decisiveness, strain, ability to overcome difficulties, enjoyment, depression, confidence, worthlessness and happiness; the maximum score is 12, with scores over 2 indicating the first stage of psychological ill health and scores over 4 suggesting more serious disturbance. The HSE has a self-completion section which includes both the GHQ12 questions and a series of seven questions concerning the perceived quality of social support available (see Appendix E).

Class was based on each individual's previous occupation (or current for those still employed), grouped into six socioeconomic categories (SECs), with a further category for those who had never been employed (see Appendix A for SEC grouping). No information on income is available in the HSE but a PDI summarising the material resources available to individuals was constructed (see Appendix A).

Diet quality: effects of age, gender, living arrangements and structural/material position

In order to examine how far variation in the quality of older people's diet is associated with health inequalities by class and gender (Ginn, Arber and Cooper, 1997), the diet score is analysed according to the social circumstances and structural position of men and women.

For the sample of individuals aged 55 and over, diet scores ranged from –19 to +18, with a mean value of 0.32. A large negative score indicates an unhealthy diet, high in sugar, cakes, biscuits, sweets, salt and saturated fats and low in fruit, vegetables, pulses, and fibre-rich foods (see Appendix D).

The quality of diet showed a linear decline with age group, for both men and women. Older women's diet was much better than older men's in each age group, with a smaller gender difference over age 80 (Figure 6.1). For example, among those aged 55–64, women had an average score of over 2, compared with zero for men. Among those aged over 80, diets were much poorer, women having an average score of –1.7 and men –2.6.

As expected, those who were married had a better diet than those who were widowed or single, and women's diets were better than men's within each marital status category (Figure 6.2). For men, the effect of marriage persisted after controlling for age group, suggesting that having a wife promotes better shopping, cooking and eating practices. Among women, those who were single had better diets than those who were widowed. Perhaps surprisingly, older men and women who were divorced or separated had at least as good a diet as the married group, while cohabiting men and women had relatively poor diets; however, the numbers in these categories were small (n = 83), making the diet scores less reliable than for other groups. Single and widowed men had the most unhealthy diets.

In order to investigate the effect of living arrangements, the widowed and single groups were subdivided into those living alone and those living with others in their household. This indicated that among older men, those who were single but living with other(s) had as good a

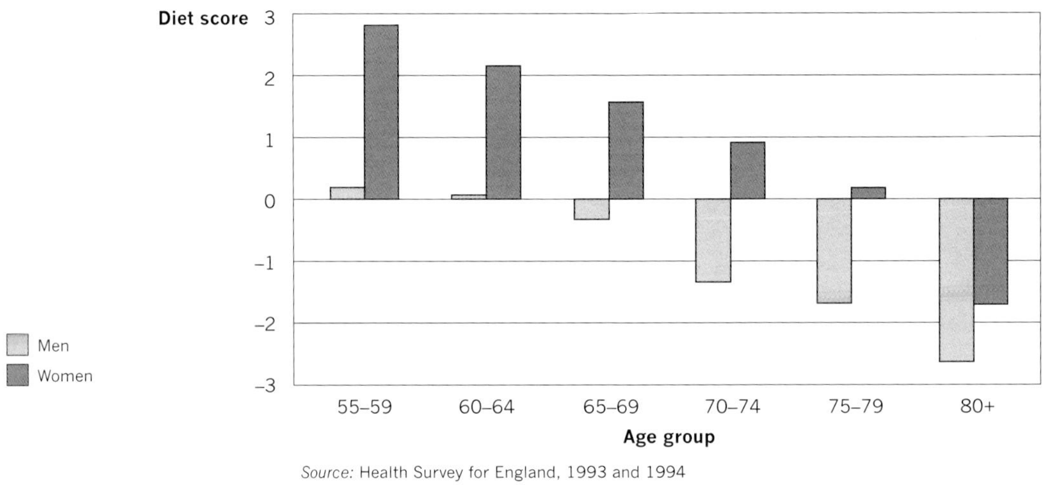

Fig. 6.1. Diet scores by age group: men and women aged 55+

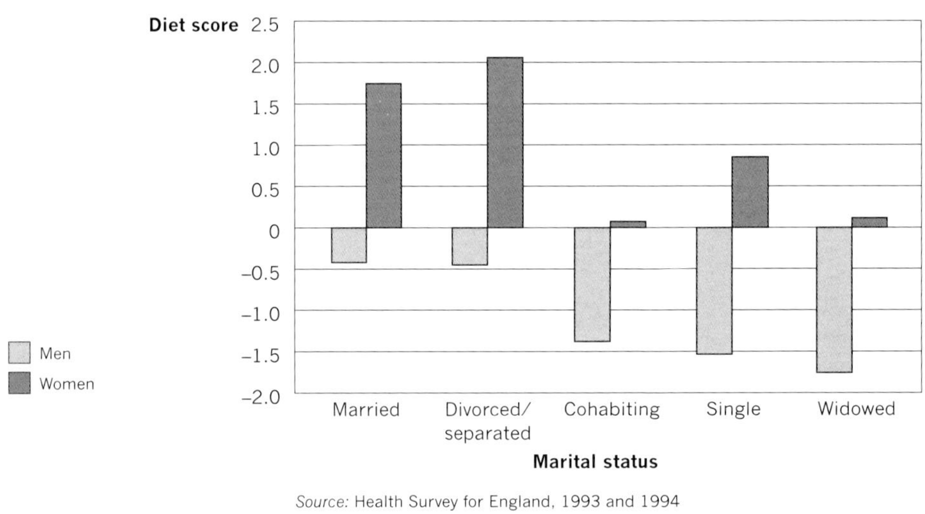

Fig. 6.2. Diet scores for men and women aged 55+ by marital status

diet as those who were married, whereas single men living alone had a much poorer diet.

Social support and psychosocial health (GHQ12 score) were only weakly associated with diet quality. Diets were poorer for older men and women with a GHQ12 score over 4, which indicates depression, and where there was a severe lack of social support (Figures 6.3 and 6.4). Analysis of stress levels confirmed that stress was higher among older people living in deprived conditions. These results are consistent with the hypothesis that deprivation may give rise to comfort eating to compensate for stress or lack of close relationships, although this is not

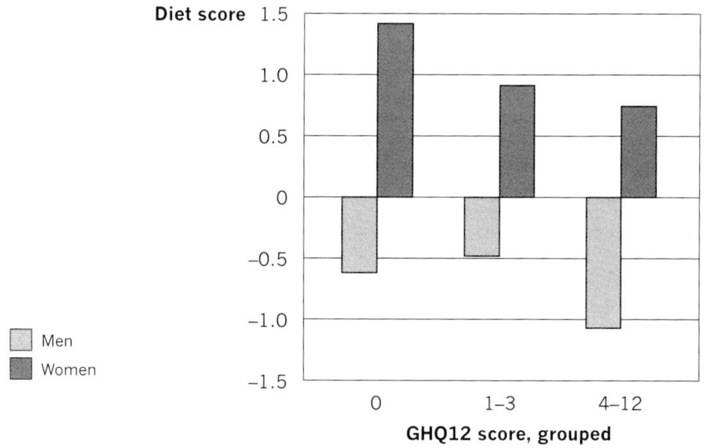

Source: Health Survey for England, 1993 and 1994

Fig. 6.3. Diet scores by psychosocial health: men and women aged 55+

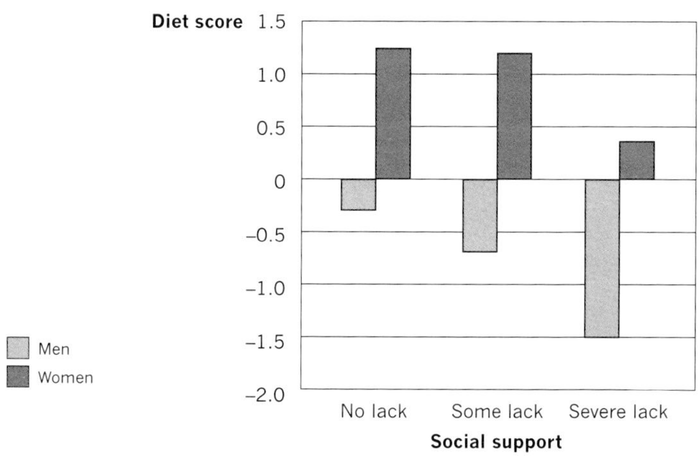

Source: Health Survey for England, 1993 and 1994

Fig. 6.4. Diet scores by social support: men and women aged 55+

a strong effect and multivariate analysis of the determinants of diet is necessary to control for the effects of age and ill health on diet.

Both class, based on the individual's previous occupation, and material deprivation, measured by the PDI, were strongly associated with diet scores (Figures 6.5 and 6.6). The striking gradients in the diet scores of older men and women by class and current availablity of material resources mirror the familiar gradients in mortality by class and point to the possible role of diet in explaining class-related health inequalities, even among older people.

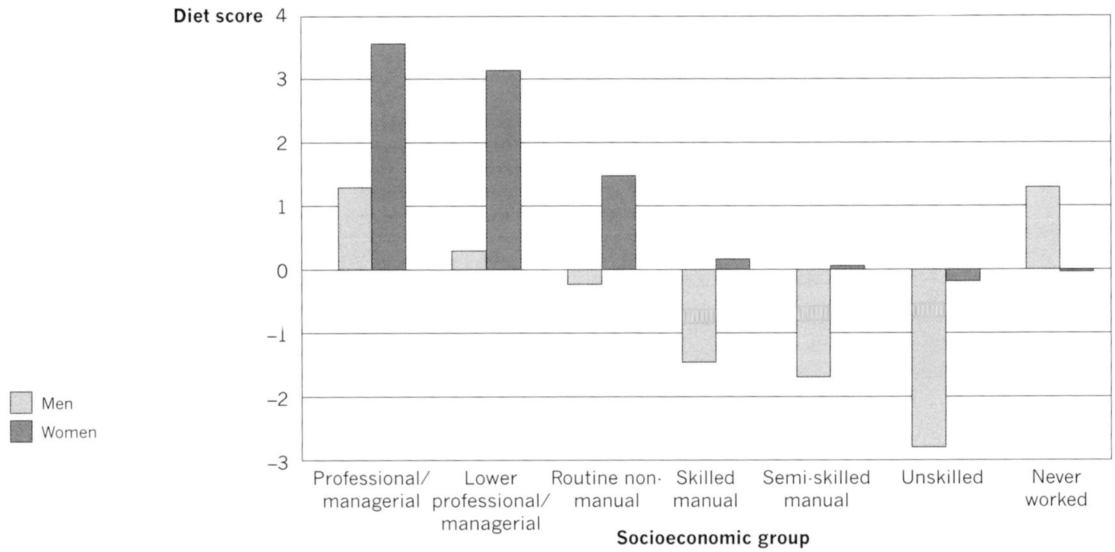

Source: Health Survey for England, 1993 and 1994

Fig. 6.5. Diet scores for men and women by socioeconomic group, aged 55+

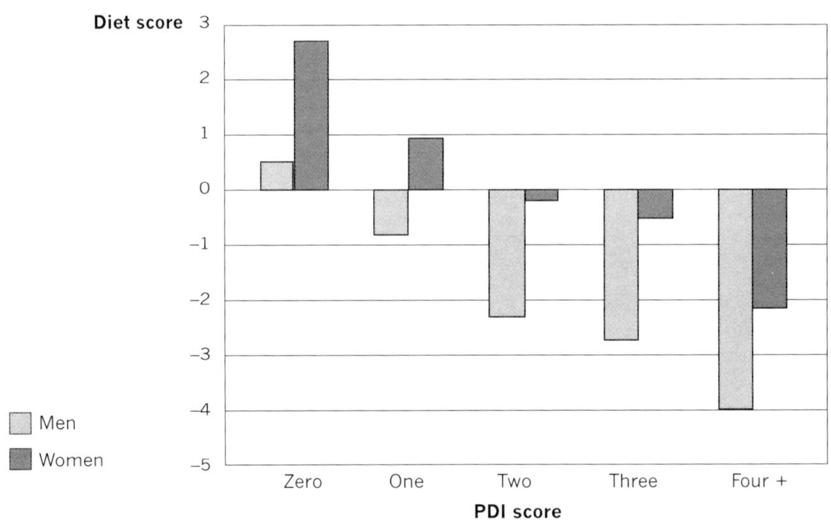

Source: Health Survey for England, 1993 and 1994

Fig. 6.6. Diet scores for men and women by personal deprivation index (PDI), aged 55+

Multivariate analysis

The independent effects of all the above variables on diet quality can best be determined using logistic regression analysis, with diet score as the dependent variable, dichotomised as above or below zero (which is close to the mean score). Tables 6.1 (for men) and 6.2 (for women)

Table 6.1. Odds ratios of having a poorer than average diet: men aged 55+

	Model 1	Model 2	Model 3	Model 4	Model 5
Age	†††	†††	†††	†††	†††
55–59	1.00	1.00	1.00	1.00	1.00
60–64	1.03	1.02	1.02	1.03	1.02
65–69	1.19	1.17	1.18	1.18	1.17
70–74	1.42 ***	1.35 **	1.35 **	1.36 **	1.35 **
75–79	1.85 ***	1.69 ***	1.69 ***	1.70 ***	1.70 ***
80+	2.51 ***	2.15 ***	2.22 ***	2.23 ***	2.24 ***
General health	ns	ns	ns	ns	ns
Very good/good	1.00	1.00	1.00	1.00	1.00
Fair	1.14	1.07	1.07	1.05	1.07
Bad	1.42 *	1.20	1.21	1.18	1.21
Very bad	1.07	0.91	0.89	0.89	0.90
Chronic illness	†††	†††	†††	†††	†††
No long-standing illness	1.00	1.00	1.00	1.00	1.00
Long-standing illness	0.72 ***	0.72 ***	0.72 ***	0.72 ***	0.73 ***
Socioeconomic category	†††	†††	†††	†††	†††
Professional/managerial	1.00	1.00	1.00	1.00	1.00
Lower prof./managerial	1.32 **	1.27 *	1.27 *	1.27 *	1.27 *
Routine non-manual	1.45 **	1.38 *	1.36 *	1.37 *	1.36 *
Skilled manual	2.26 ***	1.95 ***	1.93 ***	1.92 ***	1.92 ***
Semi-skilled manual	2.47 ***	1.92 ***	1.89 ***	1.88 ***	1.88 ***
Unskilled	4.06 ***	2.91 ***	2.91 ***	2.93 ***	2.92 ***
PDI score		†††	†††	†††	†††
0		1.00	1.00	1.00	1.00
1		1.25 **	1.28 **	1.28 **	1.28 **
2		1.73 ***	1.81 ***	1.80 ***	1.80 ***
3		1.87 ***	2.00 ***	1.99 ***	1.98 ***
4+		3.30 ***	3.71 ***	3.65 ***	3.65 ***
Living arrangements			ns	ns	†
Married			1.00	1.00	1.00
Co-habiting			0.94	0.93	0.92
Single, with others			0.71	0.68	0.69
Widowed, with others			1.43	1.42	1.41
Divorced/separated			0.70 *	0.68*	0.68 *
Single, lone			1.02	0.96	0.95
Widowed, lone			0.80	0.79	0.80
Social support				††	†
No lack of social support				1.00	1.00
Some lack of social support				1.10	1.11
Severe lack of social support				1.29 *	1.30 **
Psychosocial health (GHQ12 score)					ns
0					1.00
1–3					0.89
4–12 (Depressed)					0.99
N =	5908				
Δ –2LLR	248.9	65.0	13.0	8.0	2.1
Δ df	15	4	6	2	2

Statistical significance of variable in the model: ns non-significant; † $P < 0.05$; ††$P < 0.01$; ††† $P < 0.001$.
Statistical significance of difference from the reference category: * $P < 0.05$; ** $P < 0.01$; *** $P < 0.001$.
Source: Health Survey for England, 1993 and 1994

Table 6.2. Odds ratios of having a poorer than average diet: women aged 55+

	Model 1	Model 2	Model 3	Model 4	Model 5
Age	†††	†††	†††	†††	†††
55–59	1.00	1.00	1.00	1.00	1.00
60–64	1.10	1.05	1.04	1.04	1.04
65–69	1.19	1.11	1.12	1.12	1.12
70–74	1.50 ***	1.33 **	1.35 **	1.35 **	1.36 **
75–79	1.80 ***	1.52 ***	1.56 ***	1.57 ***	1.56 ***
80+	3.22 ***	2.54 ***	2.66 ***	2.66 ***	2.67 ***
General health	†††	††	†	†	†
Very good/good	1.00	1.00	1.00	1.00	1.00
Fair	1.27 ***	1.20 **	1.18 *	1.18 *	1.16 *
Bad	1.38 **	1.24	1.22	1.21	1.18
Very bad	2.08 ***	1.80 **	1.75 *	1.72 *	1.69 *
Chronic illness	†††	†††	†††	†††	†††
No long-standing illness	1.00	1.00	1.00	1.00	1.00
Long-standing illness	0.72 ***	0.71 ***	0.71 ***	0.71 ***	0.71 ***
Socioeconomic category	†††	†††	†††	†††	†††
Professional/managerial	1.00	1.00	1.00	1.00	1.00
Lower Prof/managerial	1.23	1.21	1.18	1.18	1.18
Routine non-manual	1.86 ***	1.76 **	1.68 **	1.68 **	1.69 **
Skilled manual	2.42 ***	2.06 ***	1.94 ***	1.94 ***	1.95 ***
Semi-skilled manual	2.70 ***	2.27 ***	2.14 ***	2.14 ***	2.14 ***
Unskilled	2.99 ***	2.35 ***	2.17 **	2.17 ***	2.18 ***
Never worked	2.11 ***	1.96 **	1.83 **	1.83 **	1.83 **
PDI score		†††	†††	†††	†††
0		1.00	1.00	1.00	1.00
1		1.35 ***	1.41 ***	1.41 ***	1.40 ***
2		1.61 ***	1.75 ***	1.74 ***	1.74 ***
3		1.79 ***	1.98 ***	1.98 ***	1.97 ***
4 +		2.63 ***	2.93 ***	2.92 ***	2.91 ***
Living arrangements			††	††	††
Married			1.00	1.00	1.00
Co-habiting			1.75	1.74	1.74
Single, with others			0.98	0.98	0.98
Widowed, with others			1.30 *	1.30 *	1.30 *
Divorced/separated			0.79	0.79	0.79
Single, lone			0.74 *	0.73 *	0.73 *
Widowed, lone			0.84	0.84 *	0.84 *
Social support				ns	ns
No lack of social support				1.00	1.00
Some lack of social support				0.98	0.97
Severe lack of social support				1.11	1.09
Psycho-social health (GHQ12 score)					ns
Zero					1.00
1–3					1.09
4–12 (Depressed)					1.06
N =	7475				
Δ LLR	370.6	68.3	20.6	1.7	1.6
Δ df	15	4	6	2	2

Statistical significance of variable in the model: ns non significant; † $P < 0.05$; ††$P < 0.01$; ††† $P < 0.001$.
Statistical significance of difference from the reference category: * $P < 0.05$; ** $P < 0.01$; *** $P < 0.001$.
Source: Health Survey for England, 1993 and 1994

present a series of logical regression models in which age group, self-assessed general health, chronic illness and class are all included, while PDI score, living arrangements, social support and GHQ12 score are added successively. This shows the effect of each added variable on the previous model.

The models for older men (see Table 6.1) show that all the variables except psychosocial health (GHQ12 score) were significantly associated with a poorer than average diet, although the effects of social support and living arrangements were weak after taking account of all other factors (see Model 5). The odds ratios of having a poorer than average diet increased with age but were reduced for those with chronic illness; this may reflect, for example, low-sugar diets among those with diabetes and low consumption of fats in response to medical advice among those with a heart condition.

Class was strongly associated with diet; for example, men previously in an unskilled occupation had odds of a poorer than average diet which were four times higher than the odds for men in the professional/managerial group, the reference category (Model 1). The effect of class on diet remained when material resources, as indicated by the PDI score, was added to the model, although it was somewhat reduced; thus low class and deprivation each had strong, and mainly separate, adverse effects on diet, reflecting respectively the influences of long-term disadvantage in the social structure and of current lack of material resources. Marital status and living arrangements had only a weak effect on men's diet, but a severe lack of social support was associated with raised odds of having a worse than average diet; this may indicate a tendency to self-neglect by older men who felt they lacked close supportive relationships.

Turning to the factors influencing older women's diets (Table 6.2), the effects of age group, general health and chronic illness were similar to those for men. The effects of class and deprivation on diet were slightly weaker than for men, while the effect of living arrangements was stronger. Widows and single women living alone had lower odds of a poor diet compared with married women; in contrast, widows living with others had a higher likelihood of a poor diet. These results may reflect greater control over their diet among women living alone compared with those who shared meals with others.

We next analyse the second aspect of health behaviour – current cigarette smoking – in order to ascertain whether there is a similar pattern of relationships with social and structural factors.

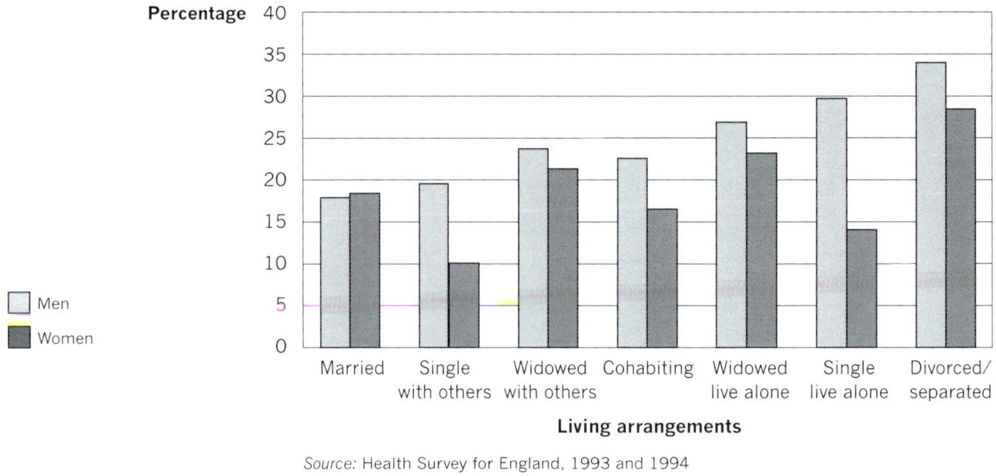

Fig. 6.7. Percentage who are current cigarette smokers by living arrangements: men and women aged 55+

Current cigarette smoking: effects of age, gender, living arrangements and structural/material position

A detailed discussion of the socioeconomic and other factors associated with current smoking among older people has been provided in Chapter 3, based on data from the 1992 and 1994 GHS. As shown in that chapter, the proportion of older men and women who smoked cigarettes was lower in each successive age group. Although women were less likely to smoke than men among all those aged 55 and over, within age groups the gender differences were very small.

This section analyses smoking in the HSE, and shows that the proportions who smoked varied with marital status and living arrangements, with a different pattern for older men and women (Figure 6.7). Older men were least likely to smoke if married (under 20%) and most likely to smoke if divorced or separated (over a third). Older women, on the other hand, were least likely to smoke if single, especially if living with others (10%), and most likely to smoke if divorced or separated (28%). These results are comparable to those reported in Chapter 3.

Lack of social support and high stress, as indicated by a GHQ12 score over 4, were each associated with increased likelihood of smoking, with the effect of social support stronger for men than for women (Figures 6.8 and 6.9). This suggests that older women may be less inclined than men to use smoking as compensation for a perceived lack of a close relationship.

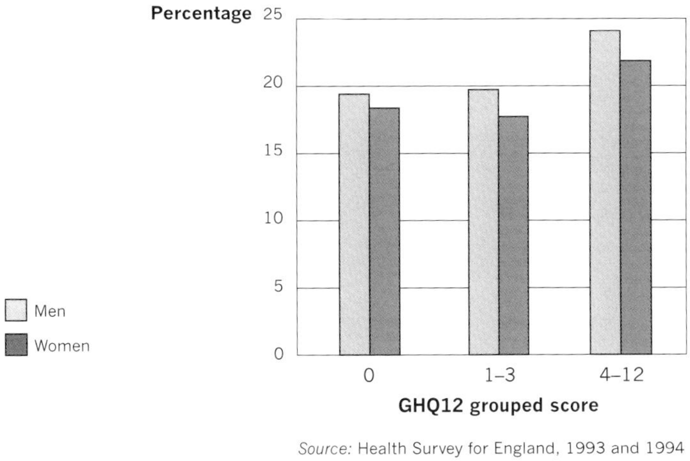

Fig. 6.8. Percentage who are current cigarette smokers by psychosocial health: men and women aged 55+

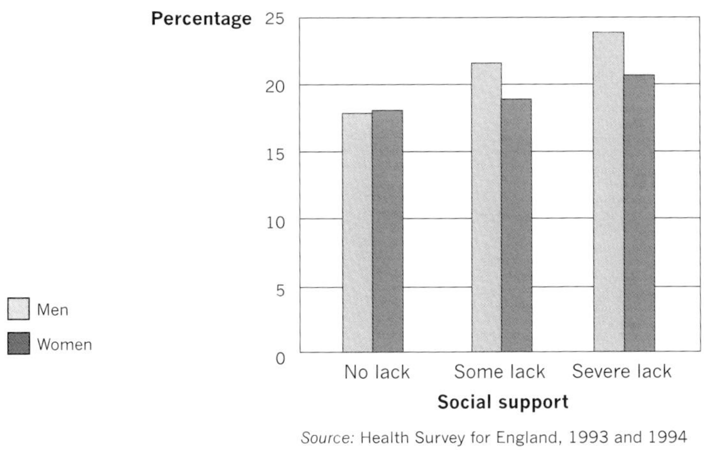

Fig. 6.9. Percentage who are current cigarette smokers by social support: men and women aged 55+

Logistic regression analysis, with current smoking as the dependent variable, enabled the separate effects of social support, psychosocial health and living arrangements, as well as structural factors, to be distinguished. Table 6.3 shows models for men. The odds of smoking declined with advancing age and were reduced for those having a chronic illness, as discussed in Chapter 3. Men assessing their general health as 'fair' or 'bad' had raised odds of smoking compared with those reporting very good/good health, but men with 'very bad' health had odds of smoking which were not significantly raised.

The association of smoking with class was modified by the inclusion of the PDI, yet remained statistically significant. Material deprivation had more effect than class on smoking. For example, in Model 2 the

Table 6.3. Odds ratios of current cigarette smoking: men aged 55+

	Model 1	Model 2	Model 3	Model 4	Model 5
Age	†††	†††	†††	†††	†††
55–59	1.00	1.00	1.00	1.00	1.00
60–64	1.01	0.99	0.99	0.99	0.99
65–69	0.95	0.91	0.88	0.89	0.88
70–74	0.66 ***	0.59 ***	0.58 ***	0.58 ***	0.58 ***
75–79	0.49 ***	0.38 ***	0.37 ***	0.37 ***	0.37 ***
80+	0.39 ***	0.27 ***	0.24 ***	0.24 ***	0.24 ***
General health	†††	††	††	††	††
Very good/good	1.00	1.00	1.00	1.00	1.00
Fair	1.54 ***	1.39 ***	1.40 ***	1.38 **	1.39
Bad	1.97 ***	1.52 **	1.51 *	1.49 *	1.50 *
Very bad	1.63	1.30	1.27	1.26	1.26
Chronic illness	†††	†††	†††	†††	†††
No long-standing illness	1.00	1.00	1.00	1.00	1.00
Long-standing illness	0.72 ***	0.72 ***	0.72 ***	0.72 ***	0.72 ***
Socioeconomic category	†††	††	†††	††	†††
Professional/managerial	1.00	1.00	1.00	1.00	1.00
Lower prof./managerial	1.22	1.12	1.12	1.12	1.12
Routine non-manual	1.50 *	1.33	1.33	1.33	1.32
Skilled manual	1.89 ***	1.42 **	1.42 **	1.42 **	1.42 **
Semi-skilled manual	2.03 ***	1.29	1.31	1.31	1.31
Unskilled	4.19 ***	2.45 ***	2.47 ***	2.47 ***	2.47 ***
PDI score		†††	†††	†††	†††
0		1.00	1.00	1.00	1.00
1		1.72 ***	1.66 ***	1.67 ***	1.67 ***
2		2.27 ***	2.14 ***	2.13 ***	2.13 ***
3		3.89 ***	3.56 ***	3.54 ***	3.54 ***
4+		3.85 ***	3.41 ***	3.40 ***	3.41 ***
Living arrangements			†	†	†
Married			1.00	1.00	1.00
Co-habiting			1.33	1.31	1.30
Single, with others			0.71	0.68	0.69
Widowed, with others			1.35	1.32	1.31
Divorced/separated			1.44 *	1.41 *	1.41 *
Single, lone			1.17	1.11	1.11
Widowed, lone			1.55 **	1.54 **	1.54 **
Social support				ns	ns
No lack of social support				1.00	1.00
Some lack of social support				1.20	1.20
Severe lack of social support				1.18	1.18
Psychosocial health (GHQ12 score)					ns
0					1.00
1–3					0.94
4–12 (depressed)					1.01
N =	4339				
Δ −2LLR	188.7	123.0	16.3	4.8	0.5
Δ df	15	4	6	2	2

Statistical significance of variable in the model: † $P < 0.05$; ††$P < 0.01$; †††$P < 0.001$.
Statistical significance of difference from the reference category: * $P < 0.05$; ** $P < 0.01$; *** $P < 0.001$.

Source: Health Survey for England, 1993 and 1994 (authors' analysis)

Table 6.4. Odds ratios of current cigarette smoking: women aged 55+

	Model 1	Model 2	Model 3	Model 4	Model 5
Age	†††	†††	†††	†††	†††
55–59	1.00	1.00	1.00	1.00	1.00
60–64	1.04	0.97	0.97	0.96	0.97
65–69	0.77 *	0.67 ***	0.67 ***	0.67 ***	0.68 ***
70–74	0.58 ***	0.46 ***	0.47 ***	0.47 ***	0.47 ***
75–79	0.44 ***	0.32 ***	0.32 ***	0.32 ***	0.32 ***
80+	0.31 ***	0.20 ***	0.20 ***	0.20 ***	0.20 ***
General health	†††	†	†	†	†
Very good/good	1.00	1.00	1.00	1.00	1.00
Fair	1.31 **	1.20 *	1.20 *	1.20 *	1.19
Bad	1.78 ***	1.52 **	1.50 **	1.49 **	1.44 *
Very bad	1.27	0.99	0.98	0.97	0.92
Chronic illness	††	†††	†††	†††	†††
No long-standing illness	1.00	1.00	1.00	1.00	1.00
Long-standing illness	0.77 ***	0.75 ***	0.74 ***	0.74 ***	0.74 ***
Socioeconomic category	†††	†††	†††	†††	†††
Professional/managerial	1.00	1.00	1.00	1.00	1.00
Lower prof. + man.	0.68	0.65 *	0.63 *	0.63 *	0.63 *
Routine non-manual	0.97	0.87	0.84	0.84	0.84
Skilled manual	1.28	0.96	0.92	0.91	0.92
Semi-skilled manual	1.26	0.93	0.89	0.89	0.89
Unskilled	1.95 **	1.29	1.21	1.21	1.21
Never worked	0.75	0.61	0.57	0.57	0.57
PDI score		†††	†††	†††	†††
0		1.00	1.00	1.00	1.00
1		1.42 ***	1.43 ***	1.42 ***	1.42 ***
2		2.18 ***	2.20 ***	2.20 ***	2.18 ***
3		2.86 ***	2.87 ***	2.87 ***	2.86 ***
4+		3.61 ***	3.63 ***	3.62 ***	3.62 ***
Living arrangements			†	†	†
Married			1.00	1.00	1.00
Cohabiting			1.12	1.13	1.12
Single, with others			0.37 **	0.37 **	0.37 **
Widowed, with others			1.27	1.27	1.27
Divorced/separated			1.11	1.11	1.10
Single, lone			0.69	0.68	0.69
Widowed, lone			1.01	1.02	1.01
Social support				ns	ns
No lack of social support				1.00	1.00
Some lack of social support				1.07	1.06
Severe lack of social support				1.06	1.05
Psycho-social health (GHQ12 score)					ns
Zero					1.00
1–3					0.93
4–12 (depressed)					1.13
N =	5293				
Δ −2LLR	218.7	110.7	15.0	0.7	2.9
Δ df	15	4	6	2	2

Statistical significance of variable in the model: † $P < 0.05$; †† $P < 0.01$; ††† $P < 0.001$.
Statistical significance of difference from the reference category: * $P < 0.05$; ** $P < 0.01$; *** $P < 0.001$.

Source: Health Survey for England, 1993 and 1994 (authors' analysis)

odds of men smoking were 3.85 times higher for those with PDI scores over 4 compared with men having a zero score. The odds for men previously employed in unskilled occupations were 2.45 times higher than for the professional/managerial group.

Living arrangements had a weak but significant effect on older men's current smoking. Divorced, separated or lone widowed men had higher odds of smoking than married men. Neither social support nor psychosocial health was significantly associated with men's likelihood of smoking, after taking account of the other variables.

The pattern of relationships for women's smoking was similar to men's in respect of age, chronic illness and general health (see Table 6.4). However, whereas smoking among men was associated with previous manual occupations, only those women previously in unskilled occupations showed a higher likelihood of smoking compared with those in the professional/managerial group (Model 1) This association between smoking and the unskilled class became non-significant once deprivation (PDI) was included in Model 2, but the overall effect of socioeconomic group on this health behaviour remained highly significant. There was some indication that women who had never been employed were less likely to smoke. As for men, smoking was strongly associated with current material deprivation. The odds of smoking for older women living in the most materially deprived circumstances were over three times higher than for the non-deprived group (the reference category).

The effect of older women's living arrangements on smoking was weak, as for men. Only single women living with others had odds of smoking which differed significantly from the reference category; these women had odds of smoking of 0.37 compared with 1.00 for married women. As for men, neither social support nor psychosocial health was associated with smoking.

Discussion and conclusions

The analysis of two aspects of health-related behaviour has shown both similarities and differences in their relationships with structural and social factors. The pattern of relationships with chronic illness, social class and material deprivation is similar for diet and smoking. However, age has opposite effects on diet and on smoking, while the effects of living arrangements and social support are somewhat different for diet and for smoking and also interact with gender.

The decline in quality of diet with advancing age may reflect poorer socioeconomic circumstances, with those of advanced age less able to afford fruit and vegetables. Also, physical difficulties in getting to the shops or in managing the tasks of preparing food constrain the diet choices available; these difficulties would tend to increase with normal ageing. However, the association of a healthier diet with younger age may also indicate better information among later cohorts as to the requirements of a healthy diet. The proportion smoking was markedly lower in older age groups. It is not clear how far this is due to selection effects, in which smokers either tend to be removed from the survey population at an earlier age through death or cease to smoke, or due to a cohort effect, with later cohorts more likely to smoke than earlier.

Women had a much healthier diet than men; but in each age group cigarette smoking was almost as likely among older women as men. Marriage and living arrangements had only weak effects on health behaviour and the effects, as expected, differed for men and women. Among men, bivariate analysis showed that marriage was associated with a healthier diet, suggesting that husbands benefit from their wives' influence in selecting and preparing meals. However, once account was taken of age, health, class and material resources, this supposed beneficial effect of marriage was no longer evident. For women, the effect of living arrangements on diet was stronger, with non-married lone women having a better diet than married. This suggests that where women have sole control of their diet, it is likely to be healthier than where catering is shared with others. For men, marriage appears to protect against smoking, with those who had previously been married more likely to smoke than married men, especially divorced, separated and widowed men living alone. For women there was no evidence of marital and living arrangements having these effects on smoking once other variables were taken into account.

Social support also differed in its effects on men's and women's diet. Whereas a severe lack of perceived social support was linked to a poorer diet among men, suggesting that men who lacked close relationships may have neglected their nutrition, women's diets bore no relationship to the level of perceived social support. Surprisingly, there was no evidence of social support influencing whether men or women smoked once socioeconomic variables had been controlled.

Stress, or poor psychosocial health, had only weak effects on diet and smoking and these disappeared after taking account of other relevant factors. Thus there is no support for the hypothesis that stress, independently of living in materially deprived living conditions, leads to health-damaging behaviour among older men and women.

A key concern of this research was to assess the relative importance of structural compared with social factors on older people's health behaviour. The structural factors, class and material resources, far outweighed all other variables except age in their effects. Class had a major influence on diet and smoking. For men, lower class was associated with both smoking and poorer diet and unskilled women had the highest rate of smoking. Material deprivation had a separate and even stronger association than class with having an unhealthy diet and with smoking for both men and women. Class and material conditions may be seen as reflecting respectively long-term social disadvantage and current material disadvantage, the latter being the more potent influence on current health behaviour.

In conclusion, social circumstances, in terms of marital status, living arrangements, perceived social support and stress, had much less impact on health behaviour compared with position in the social structure, although there is some evidence that marriage and socially supportive relationships may promote healthier behaviour among older men but not women. The pattern of effects of social and structural factors was similar in many respects for both diet and smoking, indicating that the relationships established are relevant to health-related behaviour generally.

The potential of health promotion has been highlighted by the recent claim that Alzheimer's disease may be prevented by an adequate level of folates (present mainly in certain fruits and vegetables); the implications of preventing such diseases through diet are clearly enormous, for individuals and their families as well as for society as a whole. Further research is required to illuminate the processes through which health-damaging behaviour is linked to material deprivation and low class.

7 Conclusions and recommendations

Age is a major determinant of health behaviour and health attitudes. With increasing age, men and women are less likely to eat a healthy diet and be physically active, and more likely to be fatalistic about health. This suggests a decline in health-promoting behaviour and a reduction in the propensity to view behaviour as being central to good health. However, levels of smoking and alcohol consumption decrease with advancing age, with presumed benefits to health.

Older women are less likely to smoke and drink than older men, and more likely to have a healthy diet, but levels of physical activity are much lower for women than men in all older age groups. Lifetime and cohort differences in health behaviour may account for some of these gender and age differences; older generations of women are less likely ever to have smoked and drunk alcohol, whilst later cohorts may be better informed about the requirements of a healthy diet and the value of physical exercise.

Central to our understanding of the health behaviour of older adults are three key factors: their health status, marital status and living arrangements, and socioeconomic circumstances.

Contrary to previous research, we found no strong evidence to suggest that fatalism about health in later life can be attributed to the greater prevalence of chronic illness among older people. Poor health is the main constraint on physical activity for older men and women. Chronic ill health may impose practical limitations on mobility and is likely to reduce older people's confidence and perceptions of their ability to engage in physical activity, which leads to an increasingly sedentary lifestyle. Poor physical health is associated with a poorer than average diet for men and women, but psychosocial health is not significantly related to diet after controlling for these other health measures and structural factors. Having a long-standing illness (LI) was associated with lower levels of smoking in our analyses of the HSE (Chapter 6) and the GHS (Chapter 3), but smoking was more likely among older people reporting poor general health than those in good health. These associations are likely to reflect the adverse effects of smoking on health and life expectancy as well as a tendency to quit smoking on medical grounds. Our results suggest that having a limiting long-standing illness (LLI) reduces high alcohol consumption, but that excessive drinking may be greater for older men who have any chronic illness. However, using cross-sectional data, it is impossible to interpret the direction of causation between health and smoking and drinking behaviour.

A main finding of our research is the association between the living arrangements of older people and their health-related behaviour, and how this differs for older men and women. There is clear evidence that being widowed or divorced is associated with a lack of material resources in later life, especially for older women, but differences in health behaviour persist for widowed and divorced men and women after controlling for their socioeconomic position. Older men who are divorced or widowed and living alone are most likely to have alcohol consumption above the recommended limit of 21 units per week, while the lowest levels of drinking are found among married men. In contrast, married women are most likely to have an alcohol intake above the recommended limit of 14 units per week, with much lower levels of drinking found among single and widowed older women. 'Excessive' drinking (51+ and 36+ units per week for men and women respectively) is much lower for older women than for men, and our results show that divorced/separated and single older men are most likely to drink at this health-damaging level.

As well as being more likely to have a high alcohol consumption, older men who are divorced or widowed are much more likely to smoke than married men, with heavy smoking also higher among these groups and for single men living alone. For older women too, smoking is most prevalent among those who are divorced/separated or widowed, and widows who live alone are significantly more likely than married women to be heavy smokers. Although married women have the greatest likelihood of high alcohol consumption, they are much less likely to smoke than previously married women.

In addition to the lower levels of smoking and drinking found among married older men, our results show that being married is associated with eating a healthy diet for men, although this relationship is weakened after accounting for socioeconomic differences between the married and non-married. Our results confirm that as well as being least likely to smoke and drink, single older women have a better diet than married or previously married women.

The finding that marriage is associated with positive health behaviour for older men (lower smoking, drinking and a healthier diet) suggests that a partner has an important role in monitoring men's health behaviour. Being married does not have the same beneficial effect on the health behaviour of older women, with single older women being less likely to smoke and drink and having a better diet than married women. Women who are married are most likely to have a high alcohol intake, and it may be that this aspect of their behaviour is influenced to some extent by their spouse. There is no evidence that high drinking habits continue for older women after their partner dies, since widows have lower levels of drinking than married women.

The loss of a partner through death or divorce is associated with higher levels of smoking and drinking for men and smoking for women. Marriage may have an important social and integrative function, and marital dissolution may elicit feelings of isolation and loneliness that contribute towards health-damaging behaviour. Although social support was only weakly associated with smoking and diet in comparison with structural factors, it may be that older men in particular benefit from supportive relationships within marriage. However, without longitudinal data it is not possible to establish the timing and nature of changes in smoking, drinking or diet as a consequence of a change in marital status or living arrangements among older people.

Each of the four health behaviours examined in this report (smoking, drinking, diet and physical exercise) varied according to the socioeconomic position of older men and women. Men and women in the lower social classes, those with the lowest income and those living in the most materially deprived conditions are more likely to smoke and to have an unhealthy diet than more socially advantaged older people. In addition, a lack of material resources is associated with an inactive or 'sedentary' lifestyle and lower participation in leisure activities which incur some financial cost. Alcohol consumption shows the opposite relationship, with the higher social groups more likely to drink over the recommended limit of 22 and 15 units per week (for men and women respectively) than the socially deprived. Unlike smoking, drinking appears to be most prevalent among those who can most afford it. However, our results show that excessive drinking, which is most certainly damaging to health occurs to a comparable extent among the most advantaged and the most deprived groups of older men.

The prevalence of smoking and excessive drinking among the most deprived groups is likely to diminish their economic resources still further, but these behaviours may provide an important way of coping with adverse social circumstances.

Socioeconomic factors are also important in understanding the health attitudes of older people. There is a strong association between low educational level and the tendency to be fatalistic about health, particularly for older women. Education explains fatalistic attitudes to a greater extent than other socioeconomic factors, including social class. This suggests that education reflects not only current social status but also the acquisition of important life skills, such as resourcefulness, problem-solving and the ability to respond to new information. These skills may be relevant to attitudes about the role of the individual in maintaining good health.

Implications of our findings for the health promotion of older people

Socioeconomic position, as well as age and health, affects attitudes to health and actual health behaviour. Because the oldest age groups are most likely to be in the poorest health and to live in deprived circumstances, these adverse circumstances may have a cumulative effect on health behaviour, presenting multiple barriers to a healthy lifestyle. Health behaviours are likely to be interrelated and should not be viewed in isolation, as they reflect underlying attitudes to health. For example, our results showed a strong association between smoking and drinking and suggested that older people with fatalistic attitudes are less likely to acknowledge the importance of health behaviour in promoting good health.

Concentration of smoking among the poorest and most deprived older people suggests that maintaining this health-damaging behaviour, although it will exacerbate their poor economic position, may be perceived as helping to cope with adverse social circumstances. In contrast, drinking above the recommended level is concentrated among the more affluent social groups, suggesting that alcohol is less likely to be used as a coping mechanism among those with insufficient economic resources. However, there is some suggestion that deprivation experienced by older men is associated with excessive levels of drinking. Thus the influence of material deprivation needs to be considered in health promotion initiatives geared towards smoking cessation and reduced alcohol intake among older age groups.

Any health promotion strategy to increase physical activity among older adults needs to consider the health and material circumstances of older men and women, some of whom may be without access to private transport, live in poor-quality environments or be house-bound. Appropriate levels and forms of physical activity will depend on age, health and gender, and even light activities, including slow walking, are likely to be beneficial in terms of circulation and joint flexibility. Home-based exercises, including those which can be achieved whilst sitting down could provide health benefits for the most frail among older people. In addition to the financial cost of going to leisure centres or other external venues, perceived barriers to more formal leisure activity among older people may include low levels of confidence, fear of injury, lack of available peers to go with and concerns about personal safety. Qualitative research suggests that motivation is a major obstacle to increased physical activity and poor health may further undermine the motivation of older people to engage in health-promoting behaviours, creating a vicious circle. Encouraging healthier habits at younger ages may help prevent the decline into ill health in later life.

To encourage a better-quality diet among older people from the lower socioeconomic groups, foods such as fresh fruit and vegetables need to be affordable. The past two decades have seen widening income inequality among older people, dividing those with good occupational pensions from those without (Arber and Ginn, 1991). An immediate increase in the basic state pension would substantially improve the material living standards of the least well-off and would help pay for a vitamin-rich diet.

For older people with chronic illness or without private transport, the practical difficulties in getting to the shops on a regular basis or transporting goods to home may limit their diet choices. Healthy foods therefore need to be made easily available to encourage older people to purchase these items on a regular basis.

Any effort to improve the health behaviour of older age groups must therefore acknowledge the socioeconomic environment in which older men and women live, and consider the extent to which deprivation and low income constrain choice and ability to modify health behaviour. Removal of financial barriers to improved health behaviour could help those living in disadvantaged circumstances to improve their health behaviour. For example, local authorities could provide free courses on stopping smoking and could provide nicotine patches as part of the course. Local facilities for swimming and other physical recreational activities could be made available free of charge for older people, with transport provided for those who would otherwise be unable to attend. For older people receiving meals-on-wheels, the quality of their diet could be improved by adherence to nutritional guidelines similar to those which used to apply to school catering.

The supportive relationships offered within marriage emerge as an important factor in promoting good health behaviour for older men, and the implications for health behaviour of becoming widowed or living alone in later life need to be considered in more detail. Supportive friendship networks or greater community participation may alleviate any feelings of stress or isolation among these groups of older people.

Recommendations for future research

1. Secondary analysis of the health and health-related behaviour of older people from black and minority ethnic groups

There is a lack of knowledge and understanding about the health behaviour of older people from minority ethnic groups, which was not a focus of the present project. We would recommend the analysis of additional datasets which have been specifically collected on minority ethnic groups, in particular the Fourth PSI Survey of Ethnic Minorities, 1993–4 (Nazroo, 1997). This survey interviewed 5000 adults aged 16 and over of Caribbean, Indian, Bangladeshi and Chinese origin, and also includes a white comparison sample. It contains approximately 800 people aged over 55 from ethnic minority groups.

In addition, secondary analysis could be undertaken of a combined sample of six years of the GHS (1991–6), which would yield a sample of over 1000 people aged 55 and over from minority ethnic groups. This would allow comparisons with the analyses contained in this report of all older people. Such analyses of national samples could be supplemented by analysing the 2% Sample of Anonymised Records (SAR) from the 1991 population census.

The analysis of these three datasets would complement the present research by focusing explicitly on the health needs and health promotion issues relating to older people from minority ethnic groups and how they compare with that of older white people in the UK. It would also allow an assessment of whether there are similar structural and social factors associated with poor health promotion behaviour among ethnic minority as among white older people.

2. Understanding the health behaviour of widows and widowers, and single older people

Our analysis in this report shows that a key factor influencing older people's health behaviour is their marital status, but that the way in which marital status is associated with health behaviour differs between older women and men. Older men who are widowed, single or divorced have particularly poor health behaviour, whereas this is less the case for older widowed or divorced women. Older single women have very good health behaviour, unlike older single men. Therefore a key issue is to understand how having a marital partner helps support good health behaviour for older men, and why loss of a marital partner for older women has a less detrimental effect on health behaviour than for older men.

We would suggest a qualitative study involving in-depth interviews with equal numbers of older women and men who are married, widowed, single and divorced/separated, to try to provide an in-depth understanding of what influences the various aspects of their preventive health behaviour.

3. Survey of older people's health promotion activity in three contrasting locations

There is ample evidence that living in poor material circumstances and having previously worked in a lower class occupation during working life is associated with poor health and health behaviour in later life. However, a key issue is how some older people who live in disadvantageous material circumstances in socially deprived areas manage to maintain good health and health-related behaviour, but others do not.

Three urban areas could be selected with comparable socioeconomic characteristics in terms of the income and class of residents, but which differed in terms of the 'sense of community' and other environmental characteristics, such as sense of security or fear of crime. A survey using semi-structured interviews of 200 older people in each of these three areas would allow an assessment of how the nature of the community structure and supports within the community influenced health and health promotion behaviour of older people in areas where older people live in comparable material circumstances.

4. Large-scale national survey of older people's health needs and health promotion issues

A large-scale national survey of older people's health needs and health promotion issues covering people aged 50 and over, with a double sampling fraction for people aged 65 and over was outlined in Ginn, Arber and Cooper (1997). There is an urgent need for such a survey in order to better understand the ways in which structural factors, social support, social capital and local environmental factors influence the ways in which older people can be supported in changing their health-related behaviour.

5. Longitudinal research into changes in older people's health-related behaviour

A longer term goal should be to examine the dynamics of change in older people's health-related behaviour by undertaking a longitudinal study of older people's health. This study might build on an existing national survey, for example, the HSE, and interview all people aged, say, over 60, every two years. This would allow an assessment of the dynamics of health change in later life, how changes in health-related behaviour are related to changes in health status, and the relationships between household and family change (e.g. widowhood) and changes in health-related behaviour.

Appendices

Appendix A Measurement of income, class and material resources

Socioeconomic group (SEG)

Socioeconomic group in the HEMS and GHS was based on the individual's current or last main occupation.

1 Professional and managerial
2 Routine non-manual
3 Skilled manual
4 Semi- and unskilled manual

Excluded: Never employed, inadequately described, armed forces.

Socioeconomic category (SEC)

Socioeconomic category in the HSE was based on the individual's current or last main occupation:

1 Managers/employers in large organisations, professionals
2 Managers/employers in small organisations, intermediate non-manual ancillary
3 Routine non-manual
4 Skilled manual, manual supervisory, farmers (own account)
5 Semi-skilled manual, personal service, agricultural
6 Unskilled manual
7 Never employed

Excluded: Inadequately described, armed forces.

Living arrangements

Information on marital status and household composition was combined as follows:

Married
Single, living alone
Single, living with others
Widowed, living alone
Widowed, living with others
Divorced/separated.

Income

Household income has been equivalised to take into account the number of adults in the older person's household. To create the equivalised scale, household income has been adjusted in the following way:

2 adults in household	No adjustment
1 adult in household	Divided by 0.6
3 adults in household	Divided by 1.5
4 adults in household	Divided by 2.0.

It is recognised in social security regulations that the cost of living alone is more than half the cost of living for two people; for example, the state retirement pension for a single or widowed older person is 60% of the married couple's pension. The above equivalised household income adjustment reflects this.

Personal Deprivation Index (PDI)

An indicator of the material resources available to each individual was constructed in the HSE by increasing the score by 1 for each of the following items which applied, giving a minimum PDI of 0 and a maximum of 6. Those with a PDI of 4 or more, which represents a high level of deprivation, were grouped together.

No central heating in household
No telephone in household
No car in household
Home not owned
Unemployed (rather than economically inactive)
Income Support received by anyone in household.

Educational level

This was based on the highest educational qualification obtained and collapsed into five categories as shown below:

Educational level categories

1	Higher	Degree or equivalent; teaching/other higher qualification.
2	A level	A level or equivalent
3	O level	O level/GCSE or equivalent
4	Other	CSE or equivalent; CSE ungraded
5	None	None of the above.

In Chapter 5, the highest two categories are combined.

Appendix B Measurement of attitudes, smoking and drinking

Fatalism

A measure of fatalism in HEMS was based on responses to the statement:

'Generally health is a matter of luck'

Strongly agree/agree	Fatalistic attitude
Strongly disagree/disagree/don't know	Non-fatalistic.

Amount of cigarette smoking

Individuals were grouped in the GHS and HSE according to the average number of cigarettes smoked daily:

0	Non-smoker
1–9	Light smoker
10–19	Moderate smoker
20+	Heavy smoker.

Alcohol consumption

Different measures were used for men and women, to take account of the greater physical effects of alcohol on women. One unit of alcohol is roughly equivalent to half a pint of beer or a small glass of wine or a single measure of spirits. The recommended weekly maxima, at the time the survey data was collected were 21 units per week for men and 14 units per week for women. (These thresholds were changed in 1995 to a daily limit of 3–4 units for men and 2–3 units for women.) The different levels of weekly alcohol consumption used in our analysis of the GHS and HSE data are given below:

Men	Women	Level of alcohol consumption
0 units	0 units	None
1–10	1–7	Low
11–21	8–14	Moderate
22–50	15–35	High
51+	36+	Excessive

In analyses of drinking over the recommended limit, the 'high' and 'excessive' groups were combined.

Appendix C Measurement of physical activity

Detailed information on physical activity in the previous four weeks was collected in the HSE. This report analyses four broad types of activity: recreational, domestic, gardening/DIY and walking.

1. Recreational

Respondents were asked if they had done any of the following activities in the past four weeks, for how long, how frequently and whether the activity usually involved enough effort to make them out of breath or sweaty:

Cycling/exercise bike
Exercises (e.g. press-ups, sit-ups)
Aerobics/keep fit/gymnastics/dance for fitness
Dancing (other)
Swimming
Weight training
Running/jogging
Football/rugby
Badminton/tennis
Squash
Any other sports or exercise.

In this report, only the first five activities were analysed since less than 1% of older people participated in each of the others. However, the measure of individuals' participation in *any* physical recreation includes all the activities reported.

2. Domestic work

Respondents were asked whether they had done any housework in the past four weeks, whether this included any of the following, defined as 'heavy housework' and implying at least a moderate intensity of effort, and how frequently:

Moving heavy furniture
Spring cleaning
Walking with heavy shopping (for at least 5 minutes)
Cleaning windows
Scrubbing floors with a scrubbing brush.

A new variable, *DOMWRK*, was constructed to summarise this information, with categories as follows relating to work done in the last four weeks:

No housework done
Light housework only
Heavy housework 1–2 times
Heavy housework 3–4 times
Heavy housework 5–9 times
Heavy housework over 10 times.

3. Gardening/DIY

Respondents were asked if they had done any gardening, DIY or building work in the past four weeks, whether this included any of the following, defined as 'heavy manual work' and implying a moderate intensity of effort, and how frequently:

Digging or clearing rough ground
Building in stone/bricklaying
Mowing large areas with a hand mower
Felling trees/chopping wood
Mixing/laying concrete
Moving heavy loads
Refitting a kitchen or bathroom.

A new variable, *GARDWRK*, was constructed to summarise this information, with categories as follows relating to work done in the past four weeks:

No gardening/DIY
Light gardening only
Heavy manual work 1–2 times
Heavy manual work 3–4 times
Heavy manual work 5–9 times
Heavy manual work over 10 times.

4. Walking

Respondents were asked about all the walking done over the past four weeks, including whether they had done any walks of 1 mile or more, how frequently and whether the usual pace was slow, steady, brisk or fast. Two new variables were constructed: *BRISK1* combined information on whether at least 1 mile had been walked and whether the pace was at least brisk, implying a moderate intensity of effort, and *WALK1NUM* combined information on whether at least 1 mile had been walked and the frequency of such walks.

5. Physical activity as a whole

Activity is counted as at least of 'moderate' intensity by the HSE if it includes any of the following:

Any heavy home-based work
Walking at least a mile at a brisk or fast pace
Cycling, swimming and aerobics
Dancing and exercises only if inducing sweating or breathlessness.

Activity at this intensity, which equates to a metabolic rate in which at least 5 kcal/minute are used, is considered sufficient to improve aerobic capacity for the average middle-aged man (Skelton *et al.*, 1998), although with advancing age, this level of activity represents greater effort, especially for women.

The HSE provides derived variables summarising information on each type of activity and also derived variables combining information on physical activity as a whole. Our analysis of total physical activity was based on one of the latter, *QUALACT3*, which measures the maximum intensity reached in any type of activity, whether vigorous, moderate, light or absent and the frequency of this level of activity, in the past four weeks:

Inactive/light activity (defined here as 'sedentary')
Moderate/vigorous activity 1–11 times
Moderate/vigorous activity over 12 times.

A second derived variable, *ACTLEVEL*, combined information on the maximum intensity of activity, and was used in the logistic regression analysis; the odds of the individual engaging in no more than light activity (defined here as 'sedentary') were estimated.

Appendix D Measurement of diet quality

A summary measure of diet quality, or Diet Score, was constructed from data in the HSE by applying the method devised by Dowler and Calvert (1995) of scoring positively for each recommended item consumed (indicated in (a) below), and negatively for each 'go easy' item (indicated in (b)). However, because the HSE provides much less information on diet than was available to Dowler and Calvert, the Diet Score in this report cannot be compared directly with their Healthy Diet Score.

(a) Recommended items:
bread*, cereal, vegetables*, fruit*, pulses* — scored +1
(b) 'Go easy' items:
sugar in tea/coffee, cakes*, biscuits*, sweets*, margarine/butter, cooking oil, milk, salt in cooking/at table — scored –1
(c) Neutral items — scored 0

Account was taken in scoring of the type of bread (white 0, brown +1 or wholemeal +2), type of spread (whether butter –3, margarine –2 or reduced fat spread –1), type of cereal (whether high fibre +2), type of milk (whole –1, semi-skimmed 0 or skimmed +1). Frequency of consumption was scored where available (indicated by *), from a maximum of +3 for recommended foods consumed daily to –3 for 'go easy' foods consumed daily.

Scoring is illustrated below for two hypothetical diets:

Diet A	*Score*	*Diet B*	*Score*
Skimmed milk	+1	Whole milk	–1
Oil used in cooking	–1	Oil used in cooking	–1
Low/reduced fat spread	–1	Butter used	–3
Wholemeal bread	+2	White bread	0
High fibre cereal	+2	No cereal	0
Salt added in cooking	–1	Salt added in cooking	–1
Salt at table occasionally	–1	Salt at table generally	–2
No sugar in tea	0	Sugar in tea	–3
No sugar in coffee	0	Sugar in coffee	–3
Cakes <2 days/week	–1	Cakes 2–6 days/week	–2
Biscuits <2 days/week	–1	Biscuits 2–6 days/week	–2
Sweets rarely	0	Sweets 2–6 days/week	–2
Vegetables daily	+3	Vegetables 5–6 days/week	+2
Fruit 5–6 days/week	+3	Fruit 5–6 days/week	+3
Bread daily	+3	Bread daily	+3
Diet score	+8		–12

Appendix E Measurement of social support and psychosocial health

Social support

Social support is measured in the HSE by responses (true – score 3, partly true – score 2, not true – score 1) to the following seven questions in the self-completion section.

There are people I know – amongst my family and friends – who …

1 *do things to make me happy*
2 *make me feel loved*
3 *can be relied on no matter what happens*
4 *would see that I am taken care of if I needed to be*
5 *accept me just as I am*
6 *make me feel an important part of their lives*
7 *give me support and encouragement.*

Possible scores ranged from 6 to 21, since the score was computed to allow a maximum of one item to be missing. An HSE-derived variable, PSSSCR2, grouped the scores:

21 No lack of social support
18–20 Some lack
6–17 Severe lack.

Psychosocial health

The following 12 questions were included in the self-completion section of the HSE:

Have you recently …

1 *been able to concentrate on whatever you're doing?*
2 *lost much sleep over worry?*
3 *felt you were playing a useful part in things?*
4 *felt capable of making decisions about things?*
5 *felt constantly under strain?*
6 *felt you couldn't overcome your difficulties?*
7 *been able to enjoy your normal day-to-day activities?*
8 *been able to face up to your problems?*
9 *been feeling unhappy and depressed?*
10 *been losing confidence in yourself?*
11 *been thinking of yourself as a worthless person?*
12 *been feeling reasonably happy, all things considered?*

Four categories of response were possible, indicating whether each state of mind was present and whether this was the same, more or less than usual. The HSE provides a derived variable, *GHQG2* (categories 0, 1–3 and 4–12), which was used in the analysis. The last category indicates disturbed psychosocial health, which we have referred to as stress.

References

Abella, R and Heslin, R (1984) 'Health, locus of control, values and the behaviour of family and friends: an integrated approach to understanding health behaviour', *Basic and Applied Social Psychology* **5**: 283–93.

Activity and Health Research (1992) *Allied Dunbar National Fitness Survey: Main Findings*. London: Sports Council and Health Education Authority.

Arber, S and Cooper, H (1999) 'Gender differences in health in later life: the new paradox?', *Social Science and Medicine* **48**(1): 61–76.

Arber, S and Ginn, J (1991) *Gender and Later life: A Sociological Analysis of Resources and Constraints*. London: Sage.

Arber, S and Ginn, J (1993) 'Gender and inequalities in health in later life', in M Stacey and V Olensen (eds) *Social Science and Medicine: Special Issue on Women, Men and Health* **36**(1): 33–46.

Backett, K C and Davison, C (1995) 'Lifecourse and lifestyle: the social and cultural location of health behaviours', *Social Science and Medicine* **40**(5): 629–38.

Bandura, A (1986) *Social Foundations of Thought and Action*. Engelwood Cliffs, NJ: Prentice-Hall.

Bankoff, E (1983) 'Social support and adaptation to widowhood', *Journal of Marriage and the Family* **45**: 827–39.

Barnes, G N (1979) 'Alcohol use among older persons: findings from a Western New York State general population survey', *American Geriatrics Journal* **27**(6): 244–50.

Baylor, A and Spirdoso, W (1988) 'Systematic aerobic exercise and components of reaction time in older women', *Journals of Gerontology* **43**(5): 121–6.

Becker, M H (1986) 'The tyranny of health promotion', *Public Health Reviews* **14**: 15–25.

Bennett, N, Dodd, T, Glatley, J, Freeth, S and Bolling, K (1995) *Health Survey for England 1993*. Social Survey Division OPCS. London: HMSO.

Bennett, N, Jarvis, L, Rowlands, O, Singleton, N and Haselden, L (1996) *Living in Britain: Results from the 1994 General Household Survey*.. OPCS. London: HMSO.

Berkman, L and Syme, S (1979) 'Social networks, host resistance and mortality. A nine year follow up of Alameda County residents', *American Journal of Epidemiology* **109**: 186–204.

Blane, D (1985) 'An assessment of the Black Report's "explanations" of health inequalities', *Sociology of Health and Illness* **7**(3): 423–45.

Blumenthal, J, Emery, C, Madder, D, George, L, Coleman, R, Riddle, M, McKee, D, Reasoner, J and Williams, R (1989) 'Cardiovascular and behavioural effects of aerobic exercise training on the health of older men and women', *Journal of Gerontology* **44**(5): M147–57.

Bone, M, Bebbington, A, Jagger, C, Morgan, K and Nicolaas, G (1995) *Health Expectancy and its Uses*. London: HMSO.

Bridgwood, A, Malbon, G, Lader, D and Matheson, J (1996) *Health in England 1995: What People Know, What People Think, What People Do* ONS/HEA. London: HMSO.

Brownell, K D (1991) 'Personal responsibility and control over our bodies: when expectation exceeds reality', *Health Psychology* **10**(5): 303–10.

Burrows, R and Nettleton, S (1995) 'Going against the grain: smoking and "heavy" drinking amongst the British middle classes', *Sociology of Health and Illness* **17**: 5.

Busschbach, J J V, Hessing, D J and De Charro, F T (1993) 'The utility of health at different stages of life: a quantitative approach', *Social Science and Medicine* **37**(2): 153–158.

Central Statistical Office (1996) *Social Trends, 1996 Edition*. London: HMSO.

Clark, D (1996) 'Age, socioeconomic status and exercise self-efficacy', *The Gerontologist* **36**(2): 157–64.

Clark, D, Patrick, D, Grembowski, D and Durham, M (1995) 'Socioeconomic status and exercise self-efficacy in late life', *Journal of Behavioural Medicine* **18**: 355–76.

Cohen, S and Syme, L (1985) (eds) *Social Support and Health*. New York: Academic Press.

Cohen, S and Willis, T (1985) 'Stress, social support and the buffering hypothesis', *Psychological Bulletin* **98**(2): 310–57.

Colhoun, H and Prescott-Clarke, P (eds) (1996) *Health Survey for England 1994*. London: HMSO.

Cooper, H, Arber, S, Fee, L and Ginn, J (1999) *The Influence of Social Capital and Social Support on Health: a Review and Analysis of British Data*. London: Health Education Authority.

Council of Europe (1995) *Eurofit for Adults*. Strasbourg: Council of Europe.

Cox, B, Huppert, F and Whichelow, M (1993) (eds) *The Health and Lifestyle Survey: Seven Years On*. Aldershot: Dartmouth.

Cramer, D (1993) 'Living alone, marital status, gender and health', *Journal of Community and Applied Social Psychology* **3**: 1–15.

Crawford, R (1977) 'You are dangerous to your health: the ideology and politics of victim blaming', *International Journal of Health Services* **7**: 663.

Crawford, R (1984) 'A cultural account of "health": control, release and the social body', in McKinlay, J B (ed.) *Issues in the Political Economy of Health Care*. New York: Tavistock Publications.

Davidson, K (1998) '"Women grieve, men replace" – myth or reality? Gender differences in the meanings of widowhood'. Unpublished PhD thesis, University of Surrey.

Davison, C, Frankel, S and Davey Smith, G (1992) 'The limits of lifestyle: re-assessing "fatalism" in the popular culture of illness prevention', *Social Science and Medicine* **34**(6): 675–85.

Dawes, F and Goddard, E (1997) *Smoking-Related Behaviour and Attitudes*. ONS. London: Stationery Office.

Dean, K (1989) 'Self-care components of lifestyles: the importance of gender, attitudes and the social situation', *Social Science and Medicine* **29**(2): 137–52.

Dennison, D, Dennison, K and Frank, G (1994) 'The DINE system: improving the food choices of the public', *Journal of Nutrition Education* **26**(2): 87–92.

Department of Health (1992) *The Health of the Nation: A Strategy for Health in England*. London: HMSO.

Department of Health (1994) *Report of the Advisory Group on Osteoporosis*. London: DoH.

Department of Health (1995) *Sensible Drinking: The Report of an Inter-departmental Working Group*. London: HMSO.

Department of Health (1996) *Health-Related Behaviour: An Epidemiological Overview*. Central Health Monitoring Unit. London: HMSO.

Department of Health (1998) *Our Healthier Nation: A Conduct for Health*. Cm 3852. London: Stationery Office.

Department of Health and Social Security (1980) *Inequalities in Health: Report of a Research Working Group [The Black Report]*. London: DHSS.

Doll, R (1997) 'One for the heart', *British Medical Journal* **315** (20 December): 1664–8.

Dorsett, R and Marsh, A (1998) *The Health Trap: Poverty, Smoking and Lone Parenthood*. London: Policy Studies Institute.

Dowler, E and Calvert, C (1995) *Nutrition and Diet in Lone Parent Families in London*. London: Family Policy Study Centre.

Downie, R, Fyfe, C and Tannahill, A (1992) *Health Promotion: Models and Values*. Oxford: OUP.

Edwards, K and Larson, E (1992) 'Benefits of exercise for older people', *Clinical Geriatric Medicine* **8**: 35–52.

Emery, C and Gatz, M (1990) 'Psychological and cognitive effects of an exercise programme for community-residing older adults', *Gerontologist*, 30(2): 184–8.

Fentem, P (1992) 'Exercise in prevention of disease', *British Medical Bulletin* **48**(3): 630–50.

Fentem, P, Bassey, E and Turnbull, N (1988) *The New Case for Exercise*. London: HEA.

Finch, H (1997) *Physical Activity 'at Our Age': Qualitative Research among People over the Age of 50*. London: HEA.

Fox, J and Goldblatt, P (1982) *Socio-demographic Mortality Differentials from the OPCS Longitudinal Study 1971–75*. Series LS No. 1. London: HMSO.

Fuchs, V (1979) 'Economics, health and post-industrial society', *Milbank Memorial Quarterly/Health and Society* **57**(2): 153–82.

Gibson, (1990) 'Falls in later life', in R Kane, J Grimley Evans and D Macfayden (eds) *Improving the Health of Older People: A World View*. Oxford: Oxford University Press.

Ginn, J, Arber, S and Cooper, H (1997) *Researching Older People's Health Needs and Health Promotion Issues*. London: HEA.

Glynn, R J, Bouchard, G, Locastro, J and Laird, N (1985) 'Aging and generational effects on drinking behaviors in men: results from the normative aging study', *American Journal of Public Health* **75**(12): 1413–19.

Goddard, E (1991) *Drinking in England and Wales in the Late 1980s*. OPCS. London: HMSO.

Goddard, E (1997) *Drinking: Adults' Behaviour and Knowledge*. ONS. London: Stationery Office.

Goldberg, D (1972) *The Detection of Psychiatric Illness by Questionnaire*. London: Oxford University Press.

Goldman, N, Korenman, S and Weinstein, R (1995) 'Marital status among the elderly', *Social Science and Medicine* **40**(12): 1717–30.

Graham, H (1987) 'Women's smoking and family health', *Social Science and Medicine* **25**: 47–56.

Graham, H (1993) *When Life's a Drag: Women, Smoking and Disadvantage*. London: HMSO.

Graham, H and Hunt, S (1994) 'Women's smoking and measures of women's socioeconomic status in the United Kingdom', *Health Promotion International* **9**: 81–8.

Greengross, S, Murphy, E, Quam, L, Rockon, P and Smith, R (1997) 'Aging: a subject that must be at the top of world agendas', *British Medical Journal* **315**: 1029–31.

Grossman, M (1976) 'The correlation between health and schooling', in Terleckij, N (ed.) *Household Production and Consumption*. Washington, DC: National Bureau of Economics Research, pp. 147–211.

Hall, W Flaherty, B and Homel, P (1992) 'The public perception of the risks and benefits of alcohol consumption', *Australian Journal of Public Health* **16**(1): 38–42.

Haskell, W (1997) 'Personal health benefits of exercise for older people', Research into Ageing's 21st Anniversary lecture, presented at Active for Later Life Conference, Birmingham.

Health Education Authority (1995) *Health and Lifestyles: A Survey of the UK Population*. London: HEA.

Health Education Authority (1996) 'Smoking kills 330 people every day'. (News release: SMOK/96/0011). London: HEA.

Huppert, F and Whittington, J (1993) 'Longitudinal changes in mental state and personality measures', in B Cox, F Huppert and M Whichelow (eds) *The Health and Lifestyle Survey: Seven Years On*. Aldershot: Dartmouth, chapter 8.

Isdale, D (1993) 'Arthritis', *Reviews in Clinical Gerontology* **3**: 259–80.

Jacob, T and Seilhamer, R A (1982) 'The impact on spouses and how they cope', in J Orford and J Harwin (eds) *Alcohol and the Family*. London: Croom Helm.

Jarvis, M J (1994) 'A profile of tobacco smoking', *Addiction* **89**(11): 1371–6.

Jerrome, D (1990) 'Frailty and friendship', *Journal of Cross-cultural Gerontology* **5**(1): 51–64.

King, M and Tinetti, M (1995) 'Falls in community-dwelling older persons', *American Geriatrics Society Journal* **43**: 1146–54.

Lachman, M E (1986) 'Personal control in later life: stability, change and cognitive correlates', in M M Baltes and P B Baltes (eds) (1986) *The Psychology of Control and Aging*. Hillsdale, NJ: Lawrence Erlbaum.

Lahelma, E, Rankonen, D, Berg, M A, Helakorpi, S, Prattala, R, Puska, P and Uutela, A (1997) 'Changes in health status and health behaviour among Finnish adults 1978–1993', *Scandinavian Journal of Work, Environmental Health* **23**(supp. 3): 85–90.

Langlie, J (1977) 'Social networks, health beliefs and preventive health behaviour', *Journal of Health and Social Behaviour* **18**: 244–60.

Leigh, J (1983) 'Direct and indirect effects of education on health', *Social Science and Medicine* **17**(4): 227–34.

Lewis, P A, Charny, M, Lambert, D and Coombes, J (1989) 'A fatalistic attitude to health amongst smokers in Cardiff', *Health Education Research* **4**(3): 361–5.

Lopata, H (1971) 'Widows as a minority group', *Gerontologist* **11**(2): 67–77.

McAuley, E, Lox, C and Duncan, T (1993) 'Long-term maintenance of exercise, self-efficacy and physiological change in older adults', *Journal of Gerontology: Psychological Sciences* **48**: 18–24.

Macintyre, S (1986) 'The patterning of health by social position in contemporary Britain: directions for sociological research', *Social Science and Medicine* **23**(4): 393–415.

Marcus, B and Owen, N (1992) 'Motivational readiness, self-efficacy and decision-making for exercise', *Journal of Applied Social Psychology* **22**: 3–16.

Marsh, A (1984) 'Smoking: habit or choice?', *Population Trends* **37**: 14–20.

Marsh, A and McKay, S (1994) *Poor Smokers*. London: Policy Studies Institute.

Marsh, A and Matheson, J (1983) *Smoking attitudes and behaviour*. London: HMSO.

Martin, J, Meltzer, H and Elliot, D (1988) *The Prevalence of Disability among Adults*. OPCS Surveys of Disability in Great Britain: Report 1. London: HMSO.

Meyers, A R, Goldman, E, Hingson, R, Scotch, N and Mangione, T (1981) 'Evidence for cohort or generational differences in the drinking behavior of older adults', *International Journal of Aging and Human Development* **14**(1): 31–44

Mirowsky, J (1995) 'Age and the sense of control', *Social Psychology Quarterly* **58**(1): 31–43.

Morris, J (1994) 'Exercise in the prevention of coronary heart disease: today's best buy in public health', *Medical Science Sports Exercise* **26**(7): 807–14.

Nazroo, J (1997) *The Health of Britain's Ethnic Minorities: Diversity and Disadvantage*. London: Policy Studies Institute.

Nettleton, S (1996) 'Women and the new paradigm of health and medicine', *Critical Social Policy* **16**(3): 33–53.

Office of National Statistics (1997) *Population Trends 88*. London.

Orleans, C T, Rimer, B, Cristinzio, S, Keintz, M and Fleisher, L (1991) 'A national survey of older smokers: treatment needs of a growing population', *Health Psychology* **10**(5): 343–51.

Osler, M (1993) 'Social class and health behaviour in Danish adults: a longitudinal study', *Public Health* **107**: 251–60.

Pescatello L and DiPietro, L (1993) 'Physical activities in older adults: an overview of health benefits', *Sports Medicine* **15**(6): 353–64.

Pill, R and Stott, H (1982) 'Concepts of illness causation and responsibility: some preliminary data from a sample of working class mothers', *Social Science and Medicine* **16**: 43–52.

Pill, R and Stott, H (1985) 'Choice or chance: further evidence on ideas of illness and responsibility for health', *Social Science and Medicine* **20**(10): 981–991.

Pill, R, Peters, T and Robling, M (1993) 'Factors associated with health behaviour among mothers of lower socioeconomic status: a British example', *Social Science and Medicine* **36**(9): 1137–44.

Qureshi, H (1990) 'Social support', in S Peace (ed.) *Researching Social Gerontology: Concepts, Methods and Issues*. London: Sage, pp. 32–45.

Rodin, J (1986) 'Aging and health: effects of the sense of control', *Science* **233**: 1271–6.

Rogers, R, Meyer, J and Mortel, K (1990) 'After reaching retirement age physical activity sustains cerebral perfusion and cognition', *American Geriatrics Society Journal* **38**(2): 123–8.

Royal College of General Practitioners (1986) *Alcohol: A Balanced View*. London: Royal College of General Practioners.

Sallis, J, Hovell, M, Hofstetter, C and Barrington, E (1992) 'Explanation of vigorous physical activity during two years using social learning variables', *Social Science and Medicine* **34**: 25–32.

Sidell, M (1995) *Health in Old Age: Myth, Mystery and Management*. Buckingham: Open University Press.

Skelton, D, Young, A, Walker, A and Hoinville, E (1998) *Physical Activity in Later Life: Further Analysis of the Allied Dunbar National Fitness Survey and the Health Education Authority National Survey of Activity and Health*. London: University Department of Geriatric Medicine/Royal Free Hospital School of Medicine.

Stroud, M (1998) *Survival of the Fittest*. London: Cape.

Swain, V (1993) 'Social relationships and health', in B Cox, F Huppert and M Whichelow (1993) (eds) *The Health and Lifestyle Survey: Seven Years On*. Aldershot: Dartmouth, chapter 15.

Thoits, P (1982) 'Conceptual methodological and theoretical problems in studying social support as a buffer against life stress', *Journal of Health and Social Behaviour* **23**: 145.

Townsend, J (1992) 'The burden of smoking', in M Benzeval, K Judge and M Whitehead (eds) *Tackling Inequalities in Health: An Agenda for Action*. London: Kings Fund Policy Institute.

Townsend, P, Davidson, N and Whitehead, M (1988) *Inequalities in Health: The Black Report and the Health Divide*. London: Penguin.

Townsend, P, Phillimore, P and Beattie, A (1988) *Health and Deprivation: Inequality and the North*. London: Croom Helm.

Uitenbroek, D, Kevekovska, A and Festchieva, N (1996) 'Health lifestyle behaviour and socio-demographic characteristics: a study of Varna, Glasgow and Edinburgh', *Social Science and Medicine* **43**(3): 367–77.

Umberson, D (1987) 'Family status and health behaviours: social control as a dimension of social integration', *Journal of Health and Social Behaviour* **28**: 306–19.

Umberson, D (1992) 'Gender, marital status and the social control of health behavior', *Social Science and Medicine* **34**(8): 907–17.

Wald, N and Nicolaides-Bouman, A (1991) *UK Smoking Statistics: Second Edition*. Wolfson Institute of Preventative Medicine. London: Oxford University Press.

Wallston, K, Wallston, B S and Derellis, R (1978) 'Development of the Multi-dimensional Health Locus of Control (MHLC) scales', *Health Education Monograph* **6**: 2.

Whichelow, M and Cox, B (1993) 'Alterations in smoking patterns', in B Cox, F Huppert, and M Whichelow (1993) (eds) *The Health and Lifestyle Survey: Seven Years On*. Aldershot: Dartmouth, chapter 12.

White, C (1997) 'Older smokers are left out of antismoking policies', *British Medical Journal* **7115**(315): 1035–8 .

Wilkinson, R G (1996) *Unhealthy Societies*. London: Blackwell.

Williams, D (1990) 'Socioeconomic differentials in health: a review and redirection', *Social Psychology Quarterly* **53**(2): 81–99.

World Health Organization (1992) *Approaches to Stress Management in the Community Setting*. Report on a WHO consultation. Copenhagen: WHO Regional Office for Europe.

World Health Organization (1995) *Epidemiology and Prevention of Cardiovascular Disease in Older People*. Geneva: WHO.

Wyke, S and Ford, G (1992) 'Competing explanations for associations between marital status and health', *Social Science and Medicine* **34**(5): 523–32.